KEYTRUDA

The Key to Immune System Supercharge Against Cancer

By

Brain T. Anderson

TABLE OF CONTENTS

CHAPTER 1
Immunotherapy's Promise"

For patients battling different types of cancer, immunotherapy is a novel approach that is bringing new hope and a different perspective. In this chapter, we explore the amazing promise that immunotherapy—specifically, Keytruda—brings to the forefront of cancer care.

Realizing the Potential of the Immune System:
The concept of immunotherapy is based on the notion that the immune system of the human body can be used to fight cancer. As opposed to conventional treatments such as chemotherapy, which target cancer cells directly, immunotherapy aims to strengthen the immune system itself. One such example of this strategy is Keytruda, which functions by obstructing specific mechanisms that cancer cells employ to avoid the immune system's defenses.

Individualized Care:

Personalized treatment is one of the most exciting aspects of immunotherapy; since every patient's immune system is different, therapies like Keytruda can be customized to each patient's unique immune response. This customized approach offers the potential for increased efficacy as well as fewer side effects when compared to standard treatments.

A Revolutionary Effect:
Immunotherapy holds great promise for treating a wide range of cancers; from lung and melanoma to bladder and lymphoma, the potential of Keytruda to unleash the immune system's power against cancer is changing the course of treatment for a great number of patients.

Cutting Edge Studies and Clinical Trials:
This chapter examines the scientific path that led to the development of Keytruda and other immunotherapies, highlighting the significance of continued research to realize the full potential of immunotherapy. The development of

Keytruda and other immunotherapies has been the product of rigorous research and extensive clinical trials.

Patient Verdicts:
In order to highlight the potential of immunotherapy, we would like to present moving tales of individuals whose lives have been changed by therapies such as Keytruda. These first-hand experiences demonstrate the resiliency, optimism, and revitalized spirit that immunotherapy brings to cancer patients.

We set the setting for a deeper knowledge of Keytruda and its function in boosting the immune system against cancer in "The Promise of Immunotherapy," which also provides context for appreciating the tremendous progress and hope that surround immunotherapy.

Realizing the Potential of the Immune System:
Immunotherapy is a revolutionary approach to cancer treatment. Unlike traditional therapies, which target cancer cells directly and often

cause collateral damage to healthy tissues in the process, immunotherapy makes use of the immune system's incredible potential as our body's natural defense mechanism to find and destroy cancer cells. One of the most well-known immunotherapies is Keytruda, which works by blocking specific pathways that cancer cells use to evade immune detection.

Visualize your immune system as a military force prepared to repel external threats. Cancer cells have evolved to pass for friendly soldiers, making it difficult to identify them. Keytruda serves as a tactical leader, revealing these covert dangers and enabling your immune system to identify and eliminate cancer cells. This process enables your body to combat cancer that is already present while also preventing future recurrences.

Individualized Care:
Personalized medicine is one of the most exciting aspects of immunotherapy, including Keytruda. Since every patient's immune system

is different and responds to treatment differently, immunotherapy can be customized to match each patient's unique immune response, offering a targeted and accurate approach that not only increases the likelihood of treatment success but also lowers the risk of severe side effects that are frequently associated with conventional therapies. In other words, it's a more patient-centric and effective approach.

A Revolutionary Effect:
Immunotherapy has the potential to treat a wide range of cancer types. For example, Keytruda has demonstrated remarkable efficacy against a diverse range of cancers, including bladder cancer and lymphoma, as well as deadly skin cancer melanoma, lung cancer, and other malignancies that claim countless lives annually. Such versatility suggests that immunotherapy could have a profound effect on the lives of countless patients.

Cutting Edge Studies and Clinical Trials:

In this chapter, we explore the scientific and historical foundations of immunotherapy, emphasizing the critical role that clinical trials play in bringing these treatments to patients. We also emphasize the significance of ongoing research, acknowledging that the promise of immunotherapy is constantly expanding as new discoveries are made. The development of immunotherapies, including Keytruda, is the product of rigorous clinical trials and scientific research. The scientific journey leading to these groundbreaking treatments involved the collaborative efforts of dedicated researchers and medical professionals.

Patient Verdicts:
To demonstrate the potential of immunotherapy, we offer moving testimonies from actual patients whose lives have been changed by treatments such as Keytruda. These first-hand testimonies attest to the optimism, fortitude, and revitalized sense of life that immunotherapy bestows upon those battling cancer. They also offer a concrete link to the possibilities of immunotherapy,

highlighting its capacity to not only prolong but also enhance life.

In "The Promise of Immunotherapy," we hope to impart a deep understanding of the paradigm shift that immunotherapy represents in the treatment of cancer. This chapter lays the groundwork for an in-depth investigation of Keytruda and its critical function in boosting the immune system's defenses against cancer. It also prepares readers to appreciate the astounding advances and the hope and optimism that immunotherapy has brought to the forefront of modern medicine.

CHAPTER 2
A Novel Approach to Cancer Therapy"

With the revolutionary potential of immunotherapy and the example of Keytruda, a new era in cancer treatment has dawned. This chapter explores the significant shifts that are taking place in the way we think about cancer, giving both patients and medical professionals greater hope and optimism.

A Change in Paradigm:
In the past, radiation therapy, chemotherapy, and surgery have been the mainstays of cancer treatment. Although these techniques have saved many lives, they frequently entail serious drawbacks and restrictions. Keytruda, the immunotherapy representative, is changing this environment by bringing in a completely new strategy. Immunotherapy uses the body's immune system to find and eliminate cancers with previously unheard-of precision, as opposed to treating cancer cells directly.

Precision Medicine's Ascent:
Precision medicine is a defining feature of this new era, and Keytruda is essential to it. Precision medicine customizes medicines to the specific genetic and molecular features of each patient's cancer, as opposed to universally applicable treatments. Keytruda is a prime illustration of the precision medicine method, as it is used selectively based on certain biomarkers.

Turning the Tide:
Patients used to frequently struggle with incapacitating side effects from cancer therapies. Immunotherapy, namely Keytruda, modifies this equilibrium by selectively targeting cancer cells while protecting healthy tissue. As a result, individuals receiving therapy have a markedly higher quality of life, which represents a major advancement in cancer care.

Complementary Therapies:

The power of combination medicines is also acknowledged in this new era. To increase Keytruda's efficacy, it is commonly used in conjunction with other medications, such as conventional therapy. These creative pairings show that the best cancer treatment may not come from a "either/or" situation but rather from a "both/and" approach that maximizes results.

An Integrated Method:
Keytruda in particular offers the potential to treat a wide variety of cancer types through immunotherapy. It has demonstrated remarkable success against a wide range of cancers, including lung, kidney, bladder, and gastrointestinal cancers in addition to melanoma and melanoma. This approach's adaptability pushes the bounds of conventional cancer treatment.

The Hope Dawn:
In this journey's second chapter, we shed light on the exciting new age in cancer treatment and emphasize the critical role that immunotherapy's

Keytruda and its peers play in it. The emergence of precision medicine, enhanced patient quality of life, the possibility of combination medicines, and the growing range of cancer treatments all contribute to the optimism around this paradigm change. We keep finding more and more amazing discoveries that are transforming the way cancer care is provided in the future as we delve deeper into this new environment.

A Change in Paradigm:
Radiation, chemotherapy, and surgery are among the harsh and frequently incapacitating treatments that have long been linked to cancer treatment. These methods have saved countless lives, but they also have a unique set of difficulties and restrictions. Immunotherapy represents a significant change in this paradigm, with Keytruda in the forefront. Immunotherapy targets and eliminates cancers by using the immune system, the body's inherent defensive mechanism, as an alternative to directly attacking cancer cells. This innovative strategy promises a transformation in the way we treat

this difficult disease by providing a more sophisticated and non-intrusive means of combating cancer.

Precision Medicine's Ascent:
Precision medicine is one of the defining characteristics of this new era in cancer treatment. One excellent example of this strategy is the use of Keytruda, which is given to patients according to certain genetic and molecular features of their cancer. This customized approach to therapy not only improves efficacy but also lowers the risk of side effects, which is a major change from the conventional one-size-fits-all approach to medication.

Turning the Tide:
In the past, individuals with cancer frequently suffered from incapacitating side effects as a result of their treatments. Immunotherapies, like as Keytruda, on the other hand, are tipping the scales by specifically attacking cancer cells while preserving healthy tissues. The quality of life for those receiving treatment is significantly

improved as a result. In the field of cancer care, it represents a significant advancement that promises improved quality of life both during and after treatment in addition to survival.

Complementary Therapies:
The potential of combination therapy is becoming more apparent in this new era. To optimize its efficacy, Keytruda is frequently used in conjunction with other medications, including conventional therapy. Combining several modalities in a synergistic way demonstrates that treating cancer may not require a "either/or" decision in the future, but rather a "both/and" approach that maximizes therapeutic results and creates new opportunities for overcoming the obstacles that cancer presents.

An Integrated Method:
Keytruda is an excellent illustration of how immunotherapy can be used to treat a variety of cancer types. It has shown remarkable efficacy against a wide range of cancers, including the

deadliest skin cancer, melanoma, the notoriously hard-to-treat lung cancer, and a growing list of malignancies including kidney, bladder, and gastrointestinal cancers. This approach's adaptability pushes the bounds of traditional thinking and creates opportunities for treating a wider range of tumors than previously believed.

The Hope Dawn:
We shed light on the exciting new era of cancer treatment in this crucial chapter, emphasizing the critical role that immunotherapy peers like Keytruda are playing. The development of combination medicines, the extension of cancer treatments treated, the emergence of precision medicine, and enhanced patient quality of life are all factors contributing to the increasing optimism surrounding this revolutionary paradigm change. As we continue to explore this changing terrain, we are revealing the incredible developments that are transforming the way cancer is treated in the future and providing new chances and hope for individuals impacted by this difficult illness.

CHAPTER 3
The Keytruda Revolution Revealed"

With the advent of Keytruda, the treatment of cancer has undergone a revolution, and this chapter aims to dissect this ground-breaking medication, illuminating its creation, mechanisms, and broad effects on cancer care.

Comprehending the Mechanisms of Keytruda
It's important to understand how Keytruda, also known as Pembrolizumab, interacts with the immune system and why it's unlike any other treatment method in oncology history in order to fully appreciate the significance of this approach. Keytruda is an amazing immunotherapy drug that works by blocking specific inhibitory pathways that cancer cells employ to evade the immune system.

From Idea to Actuality:
Years of devoted research and development have led to the realization of Keytruda as a

revolutionary cancer treatment; this chapter explores the scientific investigation and clinical trials that resulted in its approval as a life-saving therapy, emphasizing the enormous efforts of the scientific community and the perseverance needed to bring such cutting-edge treatments to patients.

Keytruda at Work:
We will discuss Keytruda's clinical applications and the cancers for which it has shown remarkable efficacy, such as non-small cell lung cancer and melanoma. Understanding the real-world effects Keytruda has had on patients, their families, and the medical professionals who administer this ground-breaking therapy is essential to fully appreciating the revolution that Keytruda represents.

The Prospect of Extended Reactions:
Among Keytruda's most amazing features is its ability to cause durable responses in certain patients. While traditional treatments often result in cancer recurrence, Keytruda has extended

patient lives, produced durable responses, and even helped some patients become cancer-free.

A Change in Oncology Paradigm:
With Keytruda, the paradigm has shifted away from treating cancer directly with chemotherapy or radiation therapy and toward using the body's own defenses to enable the immune system to identify and fight cancer. This change in approach has influenced the development of many other immunotherapies as well, all of which offer hope for a better future for cancer patients.

Revealing a More Optimistic Prospect:
This chapter reveals the revolution that is Keytruda—not just in terms of treatment outcomes, but also in terms of the newfound hope and optimism it brings to cancer patients. It is a remarkable story of human ingenuity, tenacity, and the power of science to improve the lives of people afflicted with one of the most difficult diseases in history.

This chapter lays the groundwork for a better knowledge of Keytruda and its role in influencing the direction of cancer treatment. As we examine the Keytruda revolution, we are taking you on a tour through the center of innovation in cancer care, where the boundaries of what's possible are increasing.

Comprehending the Mechanisms of Keytruda
In cancer, these checkpoints essentially act as brakes on the immune system, preventing it from attacking cancer cells effectively. Keytruda, on the other hand, releases these brakes, allowing the immune system to launch a more robust response against the cancer. This mechanism is not only clever, but it also highlights the elegance of immunotherapy, where treatment takes advantage of the body's own defenses. Keytruda works by inhibiting specific immune checkpoints, most notably the programmed cell death protein 1 (PD-1) receptor.

From Idea to Actuality:

From the initial concept of Keytruda to its practical use as a ground-breaking cancer treatment, the story of scientific progress and determination is reflected in the identification of immune checkpoints, extensive preclinical research, animal studies, and early-phase clinical trials that paved the way for larger, more comprehensive clinical trials that proved Keytruda's efficacy across a wide range of cancer types, and the FDA's approval of Keytruda for specific indications, which marked a turning point in the history of cancer treatment and gave countless patients a new lease on life.

Keytruda at Work:
Keytruda's transformative power is demonstrated by its successful applications across a number of cancer types. For example, in advanced melanoma, which was formerly thought to be incurable, Keytruda has demonstrated exceptional response rates and prolonged survival. Patients with non-small cell lung cancer, who frequently had few treatment options, have benefited greatly from Keytruda.

The therapy's application has also been successful in treating Hodgkin lymphoma, head and neck cancer, and bladder cancer, among other cancers. Examining these real-world examples highlights the profound impact of the Keytruda revolution.

The Prospect of Extended Reactions:
The most compelling feature of Keytruda is its ability to elicit durable responses; some patients experience complete, long-lasting remissions instead of just short-term ones. This promise gives patients new hope, especially those who may have previously faced a dire prognosis; the possibility of being cancer-free or managing cancer as a chronic condition has changed the narrative for many patients and their families.

A Change in Oncology Paradigm:
The Keytruda revolution represents a larger paradigm shift in oncology. While traditional treatments prioritized targeted precision and preservation of normal tissue, they frequently resulted in collateral damage to healthy tissues,

which led to severe side effects. By empowering the immune system, Keytruda and other immunotherapies mark a transformative approach that carries implications for the future of medicine as well as cancer treatment.

Revealing a More Optimistic Prospect:
This chapter is not just about the medication; it's also about the better future it opens up. It's the product of years of unrelenting research and collaboration, a testament to human ingenuity and the ability of science to rewrite the rules in the fight against cancer, and it offers hope and promise for those going through a challenging time.

The Keytruda revolution embodies the spirit of innovation and perseverance in the face of adversity, offering a beacon of hope in the fight against cancer. As we delve deeper into the Keytruda revolution, we encounter a world of possibilities that not only challenge the status quo in cancer treatment but pave the way for a more patient-centered, effective, and compassionate approach to one of the most complex health challenges of our time.

CHAPTER 4
Understanding the Function of the Immune System

In order to fully appreciate the efficacy of immunotherapy, as demonstrated by Keytruda, it is necessary to take a deep dive into the mechanisms underlying the immune system and how important it is in the fight against cancer. This chapter covers the mechanisms of the immune system in detail.

The Immune System Protecting Our Bodies:
Here, we dissect the immune system's basic function as a defender of our health and examine its ability to detect and target abnormalities in our body. The immune system is the body's natural defense mechanism, working nonstop to identify and eradicate threats like viruses, bacteria, and abnormal cells, including cancer cells.

Immune Checkpoints: The Immune System's Brakes:

Examining immune checkpoints is crucial to comprehending how immunotherapy can change the game. Checkpoints, such as programmed cell death protein 1 (PD-1) and its ligand PD-L1, act as built-in immune system brakes, allowing cancer cells to evade immune recognition and elimination. Keytruda, by blocking these checkpoints, effectively releases the brakes, enabling the immune system to identify and target cancer cells.

The Tumor Microenvironment: A Multifaceted Front in the War:

The immune system and cancer cells engage in a complex battle within the tumor microenvironment; this chapter provides insights into this dynamic interaction, explaining how cancer cells use a variety of tactics to elude immune surveillance and what happens when Keytruda steps in to tip the scales in favor of the immune system.

The Accuracy of Immunotherapy:

Precision is a defining characteristic of immunotherapy; unlike chemotherapy, which targets rapidly dividing cells in a broad manner, including healthy cells, immunotherapy targets cancer cells specifically, sparing normal tissue. This reduces collateral damage and improves the quality of life for patients receiving treatment.

What Part Biomarkers Play:

We explore the significance of biomarkers, such as PD-L1 expression, and how they help in patient selection and customized treatment plans. Biomarkers are essential indicators in the field of immunotherapy. They help determine which patients are most likely to respond to treatment.

The More Wide-ranging Effects of Immunotherapy:

Understanding these larger applications highlights the transformational nature of immunotherapy. Immunotherapy's influence goes beyond treating cancer. In this chapter, we examine how its concepts are being applied to other areas of medicine, such as organ transplantation and autoimmune illnesses.

It is a testament to the innate power of our own bodies and how science is harnessing this power to change the course of cancer treatment and, by extension, medical practice as a whole. In addition to providing a basis for understanding the efficacy of Keytruda, an understanding of the immune system's role also opens the door to appreciating the broader implications of immunotherapy.

The Immune System Protecting Our Bodies:
The immune system is a complex and dynamic network of cells, proteins, and organs that serves as the body's watchful guardian. It constantly searches for abnormalities in order to preserve homeostasis within our biological systems. When the immune system is working at its best, it recognizes and gets rid of threats, be they infections or aberrant cells like cancer. By understanding this function, one can appreciate

the enormous potential that immunotherapy, like Keytruda, unlocks.

Immune Checkpoints: The Immune System's Brakes:

Immune checkpoints are a key idea in comprehending the immune system's role in cancer treatment. Immune checkpoints are proteins that function as built-in restraints on the immune response, playing a vital role in immune balance maintenance and preventing overactivity that may result in autoimmune diseases. Cancer cells, on the other hand, take advantage of these checkpoints to evade immune detection. Keytruda intervenes by binding to the PD-1 receptor, thereby releasing the brakes and allowing the immune system to target the cancer.

The Tumor Microenvironment: A Multifaceted Front in the War:

An intricate and dynamic battle is taking place within the tumor microenvironment. Cancer cells use a variety of strategies to elude the immune system, such as secreting substances that suppress the immune system or hiding from view. It is important to understand this battlefield in order to understand how Keytruda alters the dynamics. Keytruda interferes with the tumor's defenses, making it possible for immune cells to infiltrate and attack the malignancy.

The Accuracy of Immunotherapy:
The precision of immunotherapy is a game changer in the treatment of cancer; unlike chemotherapy, which targets all rapidly dividing cells, including healthy ones, immunotherapy is highly specific; treatments like Keytruda and others target the specific features of cancer cells, sparing healthy tissue from damage; this precision lowers the burden of side effects and improves the quality of life for patients receiving treatment.

What Part Biomarkers Play:
When it comes to immunotherapy, biomarkers such as PD-L1 expression can predict a patient's likely response to treatment. This kind of personalization in medicine is revolutionary

because it allows doctors to customize treatment plans for specific patients, thereby improving the chances of a successful outcome. Biomarkers are molecular or cellular indicators that provide crucial information about a patient's disease.

The More Wide-ranging Effects of Immunotherapy:
The principles underlying immunotherapy are far from limited to cancer; in medicine, the idea of using the immune system's power is being applied to other conditions, such as organ transplantation and autoimmune diseases; this expansion suggests a future in which the immune system is used as a therapeutic tool for a wide range of conditions, revolutionizing medical practice and creating opportunities for novel treatment modalities.

To fully appreciate Keytruda's groundbreaking nature and transformative effects on cancer treatment, one must have a deep understanding of the immune system's role in cancer and how immunotherapy uses this natural defense mechanism to combat the disease. Keytruda is a journey through the complexities of our own biology and the ways in which science is shaping a brighter future for patients facing the challenges of cancer.

CHAPTER 5
The Operation Of Keytruda

This chapter focuses on explaining the science underlying Keytruda's mode of action and providing insight into how this innovative immunotherapy medication fights cancer at the cellular level.

Opening the Arsenal of the Immune System:
Keytruda's primary function is to unleash the immune system's inherent potential. The immune system, which is sometimes referred to as the body's defense mechanism, is made up of a variety of cells and proteins that are engineered to recognize and eradicate foreign objects. Keytruda works by disabling immune checkpoints that cancer cells use to evade immune detection. This is similar to giving the immune system a vital key that allows it to attack cancer more effectively and specifically.

PD-1 and PD-L1: The Principal Entities:

Programmed cell death protein 1 (PD-1) and its ligand, programmed cell death ligand 1 (PD-L1), are two essential components of Keytruda's function; we delve into the nuances of these molecules, elucidating how they function as the cornerstones of immune regulation. Cancer cells that overexpress PD-L1 are able to evade immune surveillance by effectively blinding the immune system; Keytruda, through its binding to PD-1, disrupts this interaction, shattering the shell of invisibility used by cancer cells to elude immune attack.

Getting the Immune System Started:
By releasing the brakes on the immune system, Keytruda's mechanism essentially reawakens a dormant immune response. It enables immune cells, like T cells, to identify and target cancer cells. We examine the series of events that follow this unmasking, from immune cell activation to the start of an immune attack against the malignancy.

The Selectivity's Power:

One of the main advantages of Keytruda is its selectivity; immunotherapy targets only the specific properties of cancer cells, while chemotherapy targets all rapidly dividing cells. Because of this selectivity, less harm is done to healthy tissues, which lessens the severity of side effects and enhances the patient's overall quality of life while undergoing treatment.

Extended Reactions and Sturdiness:
We discuss the factors that contribute to these durable responses, including the immune system's memory and its ongoing surveillance for potential cancer reoccurrences. The chapter emphasizes the compelling aspect of Keytruda's ability to achieve long-term responses. It is not just about shrinking tumors temporarily; in many cases, it results in sustained remissions. Some patients experience not only prolonged survival but even the possibility of a complete cure.

This chapter takes readers on a scientific voyage through the mechanism of action of Keytruda, covering everything from the natural defenses of the immune system to the molecular interactions that Keytruda breaks. By comprehending this complex process, readers are able to fully appreciate the accuracy, promise, and transformative potential of this ground-breaking immunotherapy medication in the fight against cancer.

Opening the Arsenal of the Immune System:
Liberating the immune system's inherent powers is the main purpose of Keytruda. The immune system, which is sometimes compared to a watchful army, is made up of a variety of specialized cells and proteins that cooperate to recognize and eradicate threats, whether they are infectious agents or disease-causing cells like cancer cells. Keytruda acts as a molecular master key for the immune system, opening up immune checkpoints that cancer cells use to evade immune surveillance. This action, in turn, gives the immune system the ability to launch a more potent and focused attack on cancer, enhancing the body's own defenses against the illness.

PD-1 and PD-L1: The Principal Entities:
Keytruda's function is to bind to PD-1, the receptor on immune cells, disrupt this interaction, and unfurl the cloak of invisibility that cancer cells use to evade immune detection. This allows the immune system to recognize and target these rogue cells. A deeper understanding of the fundamental players in Keytruda's mechanism is necessary. These molecules are the key players in immune regulation. Cancer cells manipulate this regulatory system by overexpressing PD-L1, effectively blinding the immune system and preventing it from recognizing and attacking them.

Getting the Immune System Started:
Keytruda's mechanism can be thought of as the reawakening of a dormant immune response. By binding to PD-1 and disabling immune checkpoints, Keytruda initiates a series of events that lead to the activation of immune cells, especially T cells, which prime them to identify cancer cells as foreign entities. These activated immune cells then launch a coordinated attack

on the cancer, ultimately resulting in the destruction of malignant cells, signifying the immune system's return to an active state, prepared to combat the disease.

The Selectivity's Power:
Among Keytruda's greatest benefits is its extraordinary selectivity. Unlike traditional therapies such as chemotherapy, which attack all rapidly dividing cells, including healthy ones, immunotherapy is extremely specific. It targets the distinct features of cancer cells while protecting healthy tissues from harm. Because of this selectivity, immunotherapy frequently leads to fewer side effects and an enhanced quality of life for patients. It also signifies a fundamental change in the way cancer is treated, emphasizing tailored and targeted interventions.

Extended Reactions and Sturdiness:
Beyond its ability to reduce tumor size in the short term, Keytruda also offers long-term responses that may even result in cures. Some patients experience not only longer survival but,

in amazing cases, the potential to become cancer-free. The chapter discusses the mechanisms underlying these durable responses, which include the immune system's memory, which enables it to recognize cancer cells and launch follow-up attacks if needed. It is the promise of long-term responses and potential cures that really distinguishes immunotherapy—which includes Keytruda—among its competitors in the field of cancer treatment.

This chapter explores the complexities of Keytruda's mechanism in order to give readers a thorough grasp of the scientific basis of this innovative immunotherapy. It also shows how this strategy is transforming cancer treatment globally by reviving and enhancing the immune system, which in turn gives patients new hope.

CHAPTER 6
Keytruda Targets and Cancer Types

This chapter highlights the tremendous versatility of Keytruda's immunotherapy and how it can improve the prognosis of a wide range of tumors by focusing on the spectrum of cancer types that it has positively affected.

Malignancy:
In the treatment of melanoma, a kind of skin cancer that can be aggressive and difficult to manage, Keytruda has shown impressive results. Many patients have experienced an extended survival period and, in some circumstances, a full remission with Keytruda, especially those with advanced stages of melanoma.

Lung cancer with non-small cells (NSCLC):
Lung cancer, particularly the most prevalent kind, non-small cell lung cancer, frequently manifests as an aggressive, late-stage illness with few curative options. Keytruda has become

a game-changer, giving patients new hope through dramatic improvements in survival and quality of life.

Occipital Cancer:
Head and neck cancers, which can affect the larynx, mouth, and throat, are infamously difficult to treat because of their close proximity to vital structures. Since Keytruda was first made available as a therapy option, patients have had significant reactions and have the possibility of better results.

Hodgkin's disease:
Keytruda has played a significant role in the field of lymphomas, specifically Hodgkin lymphoma. Durable responses, and in some cases complete remission, have been observed in patients who have relapsed or are resistant to conventional treatments, providing new hope in their fight against this cancer.

Urothelial and Bladder Cancer:

The therapy landscape for bladder and urothelial tract cancers has changed since the introduction of Keytruda, which was previously linked to few therapeutic alternatives. The medication has shown promise in producing long-lasting effects and, in certain situations, extending survival.

Cancer of the Gastric and Gastroesophageal junction:
Late-stage diagnosis presents major hurdles for stomach cancers and those affecting the junction of the esophagus and stomach. The use of Keytruda in this situation has given patients hope, as evidenced by their improved results and longer survival times.

Breast Cancer:
Treatment for advanced stages of cervical cancer, which is mostly caused by the human papillomavirus (HPV), has historically been difficult. Since Keytruda entered this market, several patients have had significant improvements in their quality of life and meaningful reactions.

Malignancies with deficient mismatch repair (dMMR) and microsatellite instability-high (MSI-H):

Due to its effectiveness in treating a subgroup of malignancies with deficient mismatch repair (dMMR) and microsatellite instability-high (MSI-H), Keytruda has drawn particular interest. These tumors, which can be located in different body areas, have distinct genetic characteristics that allow Keytruda to work particularly well on them.

The wide range of tumors that Keytruda targets is highlighted in this chapter, indicating the drug's adaptability and potential to help a large number of patients. It is evidence of the evolving field of cancer treatment, providing individuals with different types of cancer with new opportunities and rekindled hope.

Extending further

The treatment of melanoma, an aggressive type of skin cancer that frequently has a significant risk of spreading, has been transformed by Keytruda. In the past, metastatic melanoma was thought to be almost incurable, and patients had a dismal outlook. But Keytruda has significantly improved the prognosis for patients suffering from this cancer. A considerable number of patients with advanced melanoma have seen their tumors shrink significantly, and in rare instances, they have even seen total remission. This triumph highlights how Keytruda can transform an illness that was formerly fatal into a treatable one.

Lung cancer with non-small cells (NSCLC):
The disease is well-known for its late-stage detection and constrained therapy alternatives, especially for non-small cell lung cancer (NSCLC). It has always been difficult for patients with advanced NSCLC to combat this fatal illness. The paradigm of treating lung cancer has changed with the release of Keytruda. It has raised patient quality of life and survival rates, giving hope where there was none previously. This change demonstrates the

effectiveness of immunotherapy against even the most resistant cancer forms.

Occipital Cancer:
Because they are so close to important structures, head and neck cancers that affect the throat, mouth, and larynx present special difficulties. Surgical procedures frequently cause deformity and the loss of vital functions, while conventional treatments have serious side effects. With the potential to enhance outcomes and provide patients hope for meaningful responses, Keytruda has become a ground-breaking alternative. Keytruda's release signifies a significant turning point in the treatment path for those with head and neck cancer.

Hodgkin's disease:
Reed-Sternberg cells are a hallmark of Hodgkin lymphoma, which is thought to be a curable malignancy when detected early on. But the prognosis has been dismal for those who relapse or grow resistant to standard therapies. The use of Keytruda in the treatment of Hodgkin

lymphoma has been a source of great optimism. Patients who had run out of alternative treatment choices have responded well to treatment and in some cases have even obtained full remission. Keytruda's impact even reaches ailments that were thought to be incurable.

Urothelial and Bladder Cancer:
Bladder and urothelial tract cancers have long presented an obstacle for oncologists. Patients with advanced stages of these tumors had few alternatives for treatment, and their prognosis was frequently poor. Keytruda's entrance has changed everything. Patients with bladder and urothelial cancer now have renewed hope due to sustained responses, longer survival times, and the possibility of a higher quality of life.

Cancer of the Gastric and Gastroesophageal junction:
Treatment options for stomach and gastroesophageal junction cancers have previously been limited due to their frequent diagnosis in advanced stages. Since Keytruda

entered this industry, the treatment landscape has evolved. The prognosis for patients with various cancers has improved, and some have lived longer. Keytruda offers a fresh lease on life to patients suffering from stomach and gastroesophageal junction cancer, whose significance goes beyond statistical data.

Breast Cancer:
The human papillomavirus (HPV) is the main cause of cervical cancer, and it has proven to be a dangerous foe, particularly when it reaches an advanced stage. Patients with late-stage cervical cancer had few treatment options and a difficult road ahead of them until recently. With Keytruda's entry into this market, individuals afflicted by the illness now have hope. Keytruda has produced good responses in certain people, including substantial tumor shrinking and improved quality of life. This development indicates that immunotherapy may help those with cervical cancer have a better prognosis.

Malignancies with deficient mismatch repair (dMMR) and microsatellite instability-high (MSI-H):

A subgroup of tumors has distinct genetic characteristics that render them extremely sensitive to Keytruda. These characteristics include microsatellite instability-high (MSI-H) and deficient mismatch repair (dMMR). The fact that these tumors can appear in different body areas increases Keytruda's sphere of influence. Keytruda has produced amazing reactions in patients with MSI-H and dMMR tumors, resulting in long-lasting remissions and newfound hope in their fight against these genetically unique diseases.

This chapter highlights Keytruda's adaptability and highlights how it can help treat a wide variety of cancer types. It is a prime example of how tailored, targeted medicines that offer new opportunities and better outcomes for patients across the oncology spectrum have replaced the one-size-fits-all strategy in cancer treatment.

CHAPTER 7
Clinical Trials using Keytruda

Innovation and progress in medicine are largely dependent on clinical trials, and Keytruda is no different. This chapter examines how clinical trials shaped the creation, approval, and continued research and development of Keytruda.

The Critical Phases in the Development of Drugs:
Clinical trials serve as the link between scientific advancement and the provision of efficient medical care. They cover a range of phases, from early-phase studies that establish dosage and safety to late-phase trials that evaluate efficacy. Ensuring the safety and efficacy of medications such as Keytruda is largely dependent on the meticulous procedures involved in their design and execution.

Keytruda's Trailblazing Experiences:

The path of Keytruda started with innovative clinical trials that assessed its effectiveness and safety. The groundwork for later studies on different cancer types was laid by these early experiments. The outcomes of these important trials showed that patients with advanced disease may get long-lasting responses from Keytruda, including full remissions.

FDA Acceptance and Above:
In 2014, the FDA approved Keytruda for the first time to treat metastatic melanoma. This was a critical turning point in the treatment of cancer. Approvals for further cancer types, such as head and neck cancer and non-small cell lung cancer, came next. The regulatory approvals validated Keytruda's position as a game-changing treatment in the field of oncology.

Continued Research:
Following clearance, Keytruda's clinical trials have not stopped—in fact, they have only gotten bigger. These trials investigate the drug's potential in various cancer types as well as new

applications and unique combinations. In order to get even better results, Keytruda is being studied in early stages of cancer in an effort to bring the treatment schedule closer to the diagnosis.

Keytruda's Contribution to the Development of Immunotherapy
In addition to benefiting the medication itself, Keytruda's involvement in clinical trials has advanced our knowledge of immunotherapy in general. In addition to advancing Keytruda's development, these trials have opened the door for additional immunotherapies that show potential for treating ailments other than cancer.

Patient Involvement:
Patients' willingness to participate is essential to the success of clinical trials. Clinical trial participants are essential to the advancement of medical knowledge, the creation of novel medicines, and the quality of life for patients in the future. Their bravery and dedication to the advancement of medicine are priceless.

The importance of clinical trials in the creation and further research of Keytruda is emphasized in this chapter. It is evidence of the exacting scientific procedures, patients' innovative spirit, and the unwavering dedication to innovation in the fight against cancer. Keytruda's path through clinical trials is a prime example of the scientific community's cooperative efforts and the astounding advancements made in the immunotherapy sector.

The Critical Phases in the Development of Drugs:
The foundation of medication development and the key to guaranteeing the efficacy and safety of novel therapies are clinical trials. They consist of a sequence of well thought out and carried out steps, starting from the initial stages where safety and dosage are established to the later stages that evaluate the drug's effectiveness in practical situations. These trials act as the checkpoints, making sure that patient safety, ethical consideration, and scientific integrity

lead the way from laboratory discovery to patient treatment.

Keytruda's Trailblazing Experiences:
Early on in Keytruda's path, innovative clinical trials set the stage for the drug's eventual triumph. The evaluation of Keytruda's safety and capacity to trigger immune responses against cancer cells was greatly aided by these preliminary trials. They not only showed the medication's extraordinary efficacy but also heralded in a new era in cancer therapy by demonstrating the possibility of long-lasting effects. Early trial participants turned into trailblazers, helping to advance a medical discovery that would ultimately alter the cancer field.

FDA Acceptance and Above:
The FDA's approval of Keytruda marked turning points in the treatment of cancer. When the medication was first approved, advanced melanoma was thought to be almost incurable. Its scope was expanded by later approvals to

include head and neck cancer, non-small cell lung cancer, and a variety of other cancers. Every approval highlighted Keytruda's adaptability and revolutionary effect. It changed the range of treatments that patients may get and gave individuals who had run out of traditional therapy new hope.

Continued Research:
Clinical studies for Keytruda are still in progress. These studies aim to broaden the scope of what is feasible rather than only upholding the current situation. Researchers are looking at the drug's potential in earlier stages of cancer as well as new applications and innovative combinations with existing therapies. In order to achieve more favorable outcomes, the objective is to maximize patient outcomes by moving the treatment timeline closer to the point of diagnosis.

Keytruda's Contribution to the Development of Immunotherapy
Beyond its single success, Keytruda participates in clinical trials. It has helped to increase

awareness of and acceptance for immunotherapy as a ground-breaking method of managing illness. The advancements made in the Keytruda clinical trials have established a standard for the creation of other immunotherapies in the medical domain as well as in the field of cancer. It is a motivational illustration of how one innovative medical procedure can lead to the progress of the entire industry.

Patient Involvement:
Clinical trials are a monument to the tenacity and dedication of the participants, not just an exercise in scientific methodology. Patients that opt to take part in clinical trials do so bravely and frequently with unclear results, motivated by a common goal of expanding medical knowledge. They have made incalculable contributions to the creation of novel treatments. The advancements in clinical trials and the ensuing enhancements in patient care would not have been feasible without their involvement.

In the field of clinical trials, this chapter honors the unwavering dedication of investigators, the courage of subjects, and the persistent spirit of scientific advancement. It highlights the significant influence of Keytruda as a medication and as a representation of hope and development in the continuous fight against cancer and the growth of medical knowledge.

CHAPTER 8
Keytruda Success Stories from Patients

The patients who get these therapies are at the center of medical innovation and the creation of ground-breaking medications like Keytruda. This chapter highlights the practical applications of this amazing immunotherapy by presenting the motivational tales of patients whose lives have been changed by Keytruda.

Melanie's Wonder:
Melanie, a vivacious thirty-year-old lady, and her family were first devastated to learn that she had metastatic melanoma. Melanie's life took a dramatic turn when she was enrolled in a clinical trial using Keytruda, after conventional treatments had showed poor results. Her tumors started to get smaller after a few months, and she eventually had total remission. Melanie's tale serves as an example of the potential and hope that Keytruda offers to those up against overwhelming obstacles.

Robert's Story with Lung Cancer:

Robert, a retired educator, was given a late-stage non-small cell lung cancer diagnosis. He was given a dismal prognosis and told he just had a few months to live. But Keytruda turned into a ray of hope. Treatment was very effective in shrinking Robert's tumors, and he began to feel better. His scans eventually revealed fewer and smaller lesions, and he continued to spend more time with his family and even started working as a part-time teacher. His tale serves as evidence of the chance for a second chance that Keytruda provides to those suffering from advanced lung cancer.

Linda's Struggle with Uterine Cancer:

Linda, a loving grandmother, received a difficult bladder cancer diagnosis. She joined a Keytruda research trial since her options for treatment were restricted. The outcomes were remarkable. Years passed while Linda's tumors started to recede and she entered a remission. Her experience illustrates Keytruda's revolutionary potential in the treatment of bladder and urothelial cancer.

Paul's Story of Conquering Head and Neck Cancer

Paul was a father and musician whose life abruptly changed when he received a head and neck cancer diagnosis. He experienced severe adverse effects and limited success from conventional therapy. Keytruda extended a helping hand. His quality of life increased as his tumors started to react to the immunotherapy. Paul's tale demonstrates how Keytruda, when combined with surgery, can improve a patient's overall quality of life in addition to increasing survival.

Samantha's Wish for a Cure for Her Cancer:

Samantha's diagnosis of severe cervical cancer turned her world upside down. Given the dearth of viable alternatives, she enrolled in a clinical trial involving Keytruda. Samantha's tumor size significantly shrank when the medication started to take effect. Her experience shows that there is hope for better outcomes and a higher quality of life for those dealing with late-stage cervical cancer.

These patient testimonials demonstrate the significant influence Keytruda has had on people with cancer diagnoses of all kinds. They offer tangible proof of the potential, fortitude, and hope that immunotherapy—embodied by Keytruda—brings to patients and their families. Every narrative serves as a tribute to the inspirational strength of people who overcome hardship with unflinching fortitude and the revolutionary potential of scientific advancement in the field of cancer.

Melanie's Wonder:
In her thirties, Melanie was a bright young lady, full of dreams and enthusiasm. When she was told she had advanced melanoma, a particularly aggressive kind of skin cancer, her world fell apart. The outlook was dire, and there was little prospect for improvement with traditional therapies. Melanie joined a research study for

Keytruda because she was motivated to fight for her life. The outcomes were quite extraordinary. Her tumors started to diminish a few months after the medication was started. Melanie's condition worsened over time until she eventually experienced total remission. After receiving a diagnosis that seemed to be a death sentence, she was given hope for the future. Melanie's story is proof of the transformative power and hope that Keytruda may offer those who are up against seemingly insurmountable obstacles.

Robert's Story with Lung Cancer:
Robert was a retired educator who had devoted his career to instructing children. The prognosis upon receiving the diagnosis of late-stage non-small cell lung cancer was dismal. It was heartbreaking to hear that he might not have much time left. However, when Robert started using Keytruda for treatment, his narrative took an unexpected turn. His tumors showed remarkable response, progressively getting smaller and less aggressive. Robert's health

started to improve as his scans showed fewer, smaller lesions. In addition to overcoming the obstacles, he continued to spend more time with his family. He even took up teaching part-time, which is amazing and demonstrates the new lease of life that Keytruda can provide for people with advanced lung cancer.

Linda's Struggle with Uterine Cancer:
Linda, a devoted grandma, received the unsettling news that she had bladder cancer. Due to the scarcity of treatment alternatives and the pressure from her family, she chose to take part in a research trial that involved Keytruda. The outcomes were better than anticipated. Years passed while Linda's tumors started to recede and she entered a remission. Her experience highlights Keytruda's ability to change lives, especially when it comes to bladder and urothelial cancer. It represents the hope and new lease of life that Keytruda can offer patients who might not otherwise have much hope.

Paul's Story of Conquering Head and Neck Cancer

Paul was a devoted parent in addition to being a talented musician. When he was tragically diagnosed with head and neck cancer, his entire world fell apart. He experienced severe side effects from conventional therapy, which had minimal effectiveness. Keytruda extended a lifeline to him. His tumors started to respond as the immunotherapy treatment went on, and his quality of life increased. Paul's tale highlights how using Keytruda in conjunction with surgery can improve a patient's overall quality of life in addition to increasing survival. It's a tale of resiliency, optimism, and a second shot at life.

Samantha's Wish for a Cure for Her Cancer:
Samantha's life took an abrupt turn for the worst when she learned she had advanced cervical cancer. With little other viable options, she bravely chose to take part in a research trial for Keytruda. The outcomes were remarkable. As Keytruda started to work its magic, the size of the tumor significantly decreased. For others

coping with late-stage cervical cancer, Samantha's tale offers hope. It serves as an example of how better results and a higher quality of life are still possible despite a frightening diagnosis. Samantha's story exemplifies the optimism and fortitude that Keytruda offers to people and families enduring the trials associated with cancer.

These patient testimonials highlight the practical effects of Keytruda and show how this immunotherapy can significantly improve the lives of people with a variety of cancer diagnoses. They serve as living examples of the potential, fortitude, and hope that medical innovation—embodied by Keytruda—offers to patients and their loved ones. Every narrative demonstrates the deep and resilient nature of people who face hardship with unyielding bravery and the unwavering possibility of a fresh start.

CHAPTER 9
Side Effects and Safety

The accounts of people whose lives have been significantly impacted by novel treatments can be found in the annals of medical history, alongside scientific discoveries and clinical trials. This chapter highlights the incredible experiences of patients whose lives have been positively impacted by Keytruda, demonstrating the practical applications of this ground-breaking immunotherapy.

Melanie's Wonder:
Melanie, a lively thirty-year-old, was told she had metastatic melanoma, a diagnosis that would change her life forever. The prognosis was dire, and there was little chance of recovery with traditional therapies. But when Melanie signed up for a clinical trial using Keytruda, her path took an unexpected turn. Her tumors began to diminish after a few months, which was beyond

any anticipation. Melanie eventually experienced total remission. Her narrative serves as a ray of light and proof of the endless opportunities Keytruda offers people up against apparently insurmountable obstacles.

Robert's Story with Lung Cancer:
When Robert, a retired teacher, was given the news that he had advanced non-small cell lung cancer, his prognosis was dire. He was given the devastating news that he didn't have much time left to live. But his story changed when Keytruda was added to his treatment plan. His tumors showed remarkable response, reducing in size and aggression. Robert's condition started to get better as more and smaller lesions were found on subsequent scans. In addition to overcoming the obstacles, he continued to spend more time with his family. He even miraculously returned to teaching part-time, demonstrating the new lease on life that Keytruda can provide for people with metastatic lung cancer.

Linda's Struggle with Uterine Cancer:

67

Linda, a loving grandma, received the unsettling news that she had bladder cancer. She had few options for treatment, so she bravely decided to take part in a clinical trial with Keytruda. The outcomes were better than anticipated. Linda experienced a long-lasting remission as her tumors started to recede. Her experience demonstrates Keytruda's revolutionary potential, especially when it comes to bladder and urothelial cancer. It represents the rebirth and hope that Keytruda offers to those who might otherwise be faced with an uncertain future.

Paul's Story of Conquering Head and Neck Cancer

Paul was a devoted musician and a devoted father, but when he was diagnosed with head and neck cancer, his entire life fell apart. He experienced terrible adverse effects from conventional treatments, and they offered little respite. Keytruda turned become his savior. His tumors started to respond as the immunotherapy treatment went on, and his quality of life increased. Paul's tale highlights how using

Keytruda in conjunction with surgery can improve a patient's overall quality of life in addition to increasing survival. It's a tale of resiliency, optimism, and a second shot at life.

Samantha's Wish for a Cure for Her Cancer:
Samantha was diagnosed with severe cervical cancer, which was an unexpected turn in her life. With little hope for a successful outcome, she bravely chose to take part in a clinical study for Keytruda. The outcomes were really astonishing. Keytruda caused the tumor's size to significantly decrease, giving Samantha great hope. Her experience shows that there is hope for better results and a higher quality of life even in the face of a dismal diagnosis, providing comfort to those facing the difficulties of late-stage cervical cancer.

These patient testimonials capture the practical effects of Keytruda and highlight how this immunotherapy can significantly improve the lives of people with a variety of cancer diagnoses. They serve as real-life examples of the opportunity, resiliency, and hope that medical innovation—embodied by Keytruda— offers to patients and their families. Every narrative demonstrates the deep and resolute nature of people who face hardship with unflinching bravery and the enduring possibility of a new beginning in life.

Melanie's Wonder:

Melanie's tale serves as evidence of Keytruda's remarkable potential. Melanie, a lively lady in her thirties, was confronted with the sobering news that she had advanced melanoma. Melanoma is recognized for its aggressive characteristics, sparse therapeutic alternatives, and frequently dismal prognosis. Melanie decided to sign up for a Keytruda research trial because she was determined to fight for her life. The outcome was just astounding. Melanie's tumors started to diminish a few months after the treatment started. There was a significant improvement in her health. Her scans over time showed a startling realization: total remission. What had started off as a depressing diagnosis had now transformed into a future full of opportunities. Melanie's tale sheds light on the hope and limitless possibilities that Keytruda can provide for people up against the most difficult circumstances.

Robert's Story with Lung Cancer:
Robert was devastated to learn that he had late-stage non-small cell lung cancer. Robert was a retired teacher who had devoted his life to teaching. Healthcare experts gave him a dismal prognosis, suggesting that he would only have a few months to live. But once Keytruda was added to Robert's treatment regimen, his tale took an unexpected turn. His tumors showed remarkable response, progressively getting smaller and less aggressive. His scans revealed fewer and smaller lesions, which was indicative of his progress. Robert's condition began to improve—not slightly, but dramatically. In a remarkable turn of events, he triumphed against the overwhelming odds and was able to spend more time with his family. Furthermore, Robert returned to his part-time teaching position,

exemplifying the new lease on life that Keytruda offers patients with advanced lung cancer.

Linda's Struggle with Uterine Cancer:
Linda, a devoted grandma who treasured her family, received the frightening news that she had bladder cancer. Against a small number of therapy alternatives, she bravely enrolled in a clinical trial that included Keytruda. The results were not what she had anticipated. The tumors that had appeared to be intractable in Linda started to decrease. The progression did not end quickly; instead, it led to a long-lasting remission. Linda's story demonstrates how Keytruda can be a game-changer, especially when it comes to bladder and urothelial cancer. Her narrative represents optimism and a new lease on life, proving that Keytruda may provide people with the prospect of renewed hope, even those who might otherwise face a grim future.

Paul's Story of Conquering Head and Neck Cancer

Paul was a devoted parent in addition to being a talented musician. When he received the head and neck cancer diagnosis, his life unexpectedly changed. Conventional therapies yielded minimal alleviation and left him battling intense adverse reactions. Keytruda entered and offered a lifeline. Paul's tumors started to respond when the immunotherapy took effect. His quality of life increased and his health significantly improved. The combination of Keytruda and surgery turned Paul's narrative into one of resiliency, optimism, and an opportunity for a new beginning. His story serves as a moving reminder that Keytruda has the ability to improve patients' general well-being in addition to lengthening survival.

Samantha's Wish for a Cure for Her Cancer:
Samantha was diagnosed with severe cervical cancer, which was an unexpected turn in her life. Given the scarcity of viable alternatives, she bravely chose to take part in a clinical trial including Keytruda. The results exceeded everyone's expectations. Keytruda caused the

tumor's size to significantly decrease, giving Samantha great hope. Her story is a source of hope for anybody receiving a frightening diagnosis, not only those dealing with late-stage cervical cancer. Samantha's experience shows how Keytruda can transform hopelessness into fresh optimism and shows the possibility of better results and a higher quality of life.

These patient testimonials capture the practical effects of Keytruda and highlight how this immunotherapy can significantly improve the lives of people with a variety of cancer diagnoses. They serve as real-life examples of the opportunity, resiliency, and hope that medical innovation—embodied by Keytruda— offers to patients and their families. Every narrative demonstrates the deep and resolute nature of people who face hardship with unflinching bravery and the enduring possibility of a new beginning in life.

CHAPTER 10
The Continuous Evolution of Keytruda

The voyage of Keytruda is far from done; it keeps growing and changing, opening up new avenues for immunotherapy and cancer treatment. This chapter examines Keytruda's current advancements and potential futures.

Progress in Combination Treatments:
Although Keytruda has demonstrated amazing efficacy when used alone, scientists are now investigating how it can work in conjunction with other therapies. This strategy, which is also known as combination therapy, tries to increase Keytruda's efficacy by combining it with other medications or therapies. These novel combos could enhance results even more and increase the number of tumors that Keytruda can successfully treat.

Extending the Spectrum of Curable Cancers:

Keytruda was first recognized for its ability to treat particular forms of cancer. Ongoing research is expanding the range of malignancies that can be treated, nevertheless. Clinical trials are ongoing to explore Keytruda's potential in treating other cancers, providing patients with previously limited treatment options with fresh hope.

Early Intervention:
The effects of Keytruda extend beyond advanced cancer. Its function in the early stages of the disease is being intensively investigated by research. Clinicians anticipate even better results by advancing the treatment timeline closer to the time of diagnosis, which may increase the number of patients eligible for this ground-breaking immunotherapy.

Personalized Care and Precision Medicine:
Individualized treatment strategies are becoming more and more common in the field of oncology. Keytruda is essential to the precision medicine era because of its capacity to target

particular genetic markers and interactions with the immune system. To make sure that the correct patients receive the right medicine, ongoing research aims to determine which people are most likely to benefit from Keytruda.

Worldwide Availability and Cost Effectiveness:
The maker of Keytruda and medical associations are attempting to make the medication more widely available and reasonably priced. Regardless of their location or financial situation, efforts are being undertaken to guarantee that patients worldwide can take advantage of this innovative therapy.

New Developments in Long-Term Safety and Side Effect Research:
Researchers are becoming more focused on long-term safety and adverse effect management as Keytruda's use keeps growing. A major goal is making sure patients may continue their treatment with the least amount of disturbance to their daily life.

Possibilities Outside Cancer

The potential of immunotherapy goes beyond cancer. The efficacy of Keytruda and related treatments in treating other illnesses, such as autoimmune disorders, is being investigated. Novel applications in a broad spectrum of medical disorders are being made possible by ongoing research.

This chapter explores the rapidly changing field of Keytruda, emphasizing the developments, prospects, and research that will continue to influence immunotherapy and cancer treatment in the future. Keytruda is a living example of the unwavering dedication to medical science innovation, her journey one of unrelenting advancement that gives hope to others battling cancer and other illnesses.

Progress in Combination Treatments:

Due to Keytruda's exceptional effectiveness as a monotherapy, research into its potential in combination with other treatments has been made possible. One promising area of cancer treatment is the combination between Keytruda and alternative medicines. Researchers are looking into a number of combinations, such as using Keytruda in conjunction with other immunotherapies, targeted medicines, and chemotherapy. These novel strategies seek to increase Keytruda's efficacy, produce more robust responses, and expand its range of applications to include a larger variety of malignancies.

Extending the Spectrum of Curable Cancers:
When Keytruda first came to light, it was well-known for its amazing effects on a number of different cancers, such as lung cancer and melanoma. Ongoing research is aggressively attempting to increase the number of malignancies that can be treated, nevertheless. Clinical trials are investigating Keytruda's effectiveness in treating other cancers, such as uncommon cancers and cancers that were thought to be difficult to treat in the past. The intention is to give patients new hope who had

few or no options for effective treatment until recently.

Early Intervention:
Despite Keytruda's proven efficacy in treating advanced tumors, scientists are pushing the envelope by examining the drug's potential benefits in early stages of the illness. Clinicians aim to attain even better results by moving the therapy schedule closer to the diagnosis. The goal is not only to increase survival but also to perhaps find a cure. Keytruda early-stage treatment is a paradigm change in cancer care that promises improved patient outcomes.

Personalized Care and Precision Medicine:
Cancer treatment is being revolutionized by precision medicine. Keytruda is essential to this change because of its capacity to target particular genetic markers and interactions with the immune system. The goal of ongoing research is to find biomarkers and standards that may be used to determine which patients will benefit from Keytruda the most. This maximizes

the likelihood of success and minimizes needless side effects by ensuring that the appropriate treatment is given to the correct people.

Worldwide Availability and Cost Effectiveness:
The maker of Keytruda, medical institutions, and advocacy groups are working together to address affordability and accessibility concerns. Regardless of their location or financial situation, efforts are being undertaken to guarantee that patients worldwide can take advantage of this innovative therapy. This worldwide goal is being aided by projects like patient assistance programs and studies into economical production techniques.

New Developments in Long-Term Safety and Side Effect Research:
Researchers are focusing more on the long-term safety and side effect management of Keytruda as its use keeps growing. In order to give patients a treatment that they can continue with the least amount of disruption to their life, it is essential to comprehend and mitigate side

effects. Research is still being done to improve side effect reduction and quality of life for patients while undergoing therapy.

Possibilities Outside Cancer
The potential of Keytruda goes beyond treating cancer. The efficacy of immunotherapy, such as Keytruda and related treatments, in the treatment of various diseases, including autoimmune disorders, is being investigated. According to preliminary study, immunotherapies may be able to control autoimmune disorders by altering the immune system. The influence of these cutting-edge medicines is growing as novel uses in a variety of medical diseases are made possible by ongoing research.

This chapter sheds light on the dynamic environment of Keytruda's continued evolution, highlighting the astounding advancements, fresh perspectives, and current research that will continue to influence immunotherapy and cancer treatment in the future. Keytruda's journey represents unwavering advancement, giving hope to those battling cancer and other illnesses and encapsulating the unwavering dedication to innovation in the medical science profession. It serves as evidence of the persistence of medical advancement and its dedication to improving patients' quality of life everywhere.

CHAPTER 11
Immunotherapy's Promises and Difficulties

Immunotherapy has come a long way, with Keytruda serving as an example, but there are still obstacles in the way of its full potential. This chapter explores the complex trade-offs between immunotherapy's benefits and drawbacks in the context of cancer treatment.

The immunotherapy's promises:

Prolonged Survival: For many cancer patients, immunotherapy—especially with medications like Keytruda—holds the possibility of a longer survival. Some people who had short life expectancies in the past are now living much longer lives with better quality.

Less Serious Side Effects: Immunotherapy typically has less serious side effects as compared to conventional cancer therapies like chemotherapy. This improves patient comfort and makes it possible to implement treatment plans that are more successful.

Increased Treatment Options: As immunotherapy has become more widely used, there are now more options available for treatment. This not only gives patients with cancers that were previously incurable fresh hope, but it also makes customized strategies possible for improved results.

Implications for Immunotherapy:

Response Variability: Not all patients or cancer types respond well to immunotherapy. Response variability is a serious problem, and scientists are working to identify the variables that influence which patients will benefit the most from treatment.

Immunotherapy Resistance: Some tumors become immune-resistant over time. Scholars are presently investigating methods to surmount this resistance, including immune system regulation and combination medicines.

High Costs: For certain patients, the expense of immunotherapy may be a barrier to access. To meet this problem, more comprehensive insurance coverage and more affordable treatments must be developed.

Prognosis for Immunotherapy:

Personalized Treatment: Tailored treatment regimens are the key to the future of immunotherapy. Clinicians can increase the likelihood of success by customizing treatment regimens for individual patients based on the identification of certain biomarkers and genetic factors.

Combination Therapies: It is anticipated that the use of immunotherapy in conjunction with other treatments would increase in combination therapies. These strategies seek to improve results and increase immunotherapy's efficacy.

Global Access: Continued efforts will be made to make immunotherapy more affordable and accessible worldwide. By increasing access, we can make sure that all patients may take advantage of these transformative therapies, irrespective of their location or financial situation.

This chapter delves into the intricate world of immunotherapy, highlighting the obstacles that still need to be overcome as well as the successes that have already been achieved. treatment symbolizes the medical community's continued dedication to maximizing immunotherapy's promise and bringing treatment to more patients throughout the globe.

The immunotherapy's promises:

Prolonged Survival: One of immunotherapy's most alluring promises—best illustrated by Keytruda—is to prolong survival for patients with advanced, frequently aggressive cancers.

Many people who were previously given a dismal prognosis now have the chance to live far longer lives with much higher quality of life. This change in expectations is evidence of immunotherapy's revolutionary potential in the field of oncology.

Less Serious adverse Effects: Immunotherapy is known to have fewer and milder adverse effects when compared to more conventional treatments like chemotherapy. Patients will benefit from a higher quality of life throughout their course of treatment as a result. Lessening side effects also makes longer-term, more effective treatment plans possible, enabling patients to maintain a comparatively normal lifestyle while undergoing potentially life-saving medicine.

Increased Treatment alternatives: Patients now have considerably more alternatives for treatment because to the growth of immunotherapy. For many who had little or no other options, this extension represents a ray of hope. Immunotherapeutic treatments can sometimes heal tumors that were thought to be incurable before. With a greater variety of treatments available, doctors may now customize their methods for each patient, improving the likelihood of better results.

Implications for Immunotherapy:

Response Variability: Although immunotherapy has produced amazing outcomes, it is not a magic bullet that will work for every patient or every kind of cancer. Reaction variability is still a major problem. In order to pick patients more precisely, researchers are committed to figuring out what criteria predict which patients are most likely to benefit from these treatments.

Immunotherapy Resistance: Over time, certain tumors become resistant to immunotherapy, which reduces the efficacy of the treatment. In order to overcome this resistance, which is still a significant obstacle, researchers are currently investigating various approaches. In order to reestablish sensitivity to treatment, these efforts include the development of innovative immunotherapies, combination medicines, and immune system regulation strategies.

High Costs: For certain individuals, the expense of immunotherapy may be a significant barrier to access. Financial hardships may result from expensive medication and complicated treatment plans. In order to ensure that patients have fair access to these game-changing medications, healthcare stakeholders are striving to extend insurance coverage and develop more cost-effective treatments.

Prognosis for Immunotherapy:

Personalized Treatment: Tailored treatment regimens are the key to the future of immunotherapy. Clinicians can customize treatment plans to optimize effectiveness and reduce side effects by identifying unique biomarkers and genetic traits in each patient. This individualized strategy has the potential to enhance patient outcomes and quality of life.

Combination Therapies: A greater role is anticipated for combination therapies, which entail using immunotherapy in conjunction with other forms of treatment. These complementary strategies seek to solve the issue of response variability while improving immunotherapy's efficacy. Clinical professionals can increase the range of tumors that can be treated and improve patient outcomes by combining immunotherapy with chemotherapy, targeted treatments, or other immunotherapies.

Global Access: There will continue to be efforts made to make immunotherapy more affordable and accessible worldwide. In order to guarantee that patients everywhere, irrespective of their location or financial situation, can take advantage of these transformative therapies, access must be increased. This aim requires initiatives to create patient aid programs, create generic alternatives, and save expenses.

This chapter explores the complex field of immunotherapy, emphasizing both the achievements that have been made possible and the ongoing difficulties that will continue to affect cancer treatment in the future. It highlights the medical community's steadfast dedication to realizing immunotherapy's full promise and making it accessible to a growing number of patients worldwide.

CHAPTER 12
An Overview of Immunotherapy's Future

Immunotherapy holds great promise for the future and may completely change the way that cancer is treated as well as medicine in general. This chapter looks ahead, speculating on the exciting advancements that the field of immunotherapy might see in the future.

Precision Immunotherapy's Era:

Immunotherapy has the potential to lead to precision medicine, in which patient-specific medicines are carefully customized. This necessitates a thorough comprehension of the immune system, genetic, and molecular aspects of each patient's malignancy. With this knowledge, medical professionals can choose the best immunotherapies and create treatment regimens that optimize results while reducing negative effects.

93

Individualized Immunotherapy:

It is expected that immune therapy will progress beyond the use of immune checkpoint inhibitors such as Keytruda. Vaccine regimens that are customized for each patient based on the distinct antigens found in their malignancy have the potential to elicit an extremely targeted immune response. With their ability to provide tailored treatment plans and preventive measures, these vaccinations may prove to be an effective weapon in the fight against cancer.

Improved Combination Treatments:

Combination therapies, which combine immunotherapy with other modalities, will continue to develop in the future. Novel combinations, including the combination of radiation, gene treatments, and targeted medicines with immunotherapy, are being developed by researchers. To ensure better results and a greater spectrum of tumors that can be treated, the objective is to maximize the synergistic effect of various medicines.

Getting Past Resistance:

Future studies should prioritize comprehending and conquering immunotherapy resistance. Restoring the susceptibility of immunotherapy-resistant malignancies to treatment may require the application of cutting-edge techniques including modifying the tumor microenvironment and employing adaptive medicines. Immunotherapy can thereby maintain its efficacy in the face of acquired resistance.

Increasing Uses Outside of Cancer

The potential of immunotherapy goes beyond cancer. Scholars are currently investigating its effectiveness in the treatment of numerous additional illnesses, such as viral and autoimmune diseases. These treatments' capacity to modulate the immune system has the potential to revolutionize medicine by providing fresh methods for treating complicated illnesses.

Artificial Intelligence's Function:

The future of immunotherapy is anticipated to be significantly influenced by artificial intelligence (AI). Large volumes of patient data can be analyzed by AI algorithms, which assists doctors in making more precise treatment decisions. Healthcare workers can enhance patient outcomes, identify possible side effects, and anticipate treatment responses more accurately by utilizing AI.

Worldwide Availability and Cost Effectiveness:

There will be ongoing efforts to improve immunotherapy's price and accessibility on a worldwide scale. Efforts are in progress to lower treatment costs, promote international collaboration, and guarantee patients fair access to these game-changing treatments regardless of their financial situation or place of residence.

Looking ahead to immunotherapy, we see a time when tailored vaccination therapies, precision medicine, and improved combo treatments become standard practices. Immunotherapy is set to take center stage in this exciting scientific journey as the battle against cancer and other diseases continues to evolve.

Extending further

Precision Immunotherapy's Era:

Immunotherapy's future heralds a move toward precision medicine. Rather than using a one-size-fits-all strategy, medical professionals will examine the genetic, biochemical, and immune system traits of every patient in great detail. The selection of immunotherapies that are most likely to be successful for the patient's particular condition will be made possible by this thorough information. Precision immunotherapy has the potential to improve treatment outcomes while lowering the risk of side effects by precisely targeting the underlying mechanisms of the disease.

Individualized Immunotherapy:

Beyond immune checkpoint inhibitors like Keytruda, immunotherapy will advance. It is imagined that tailored vaccination therapies will be ubiquitous in the future. The vaccinations will be specifically designed to target and eliminate cancer cells with exceptional specificity, based on the distinct antigens found in each patient's malignancy. For people who are at a high risk of developing cancer, this may be used both as a preventive strategy and as a treatment. Vaccine therapies tailored to an individual's needs provide a potent weapon in the continuous fight against cancer.

Improved Combination Treatments:

Combination therapies that use immunotherapy's synergistic effects with other forms of treatment will become more prevalent in the future. Scientists are presently engaged in the development of innovative amalgamations, encompassing the combination of gene therapies, radiation therapy, and immunotherapy. The objective is to maximize the complimentary effects of various treatments in order to increase the range of cancers that can be successfully treated and possibly provide even better results. In the years to come, combination therapies may prove to be a vital component of cancer treatment.

Getting Past Resistance:

Future studies must prioritize comprehending and overcoming immunotherapy resistance. Over time, cancer cells might change and develop resistance to therapy. The goal of sophisticated methods and approaches, such as modifying the tumor microenvironment and creating adaptive therapies, is to make immunotherapy-resistant tumors susceptible to treatment again. One of the most important steps in guaranteeing the long-term efficacy of immunotherapies is the ability to overcome resistance.

Increasing Uses Outside of Cancer

The field of immunotherapy has promise outside of oncology. Scholars are presently investigating the effectiveness of these therapies in the management of numerous additional illnesses. This covers viral diseases as well as autoimmune disorders, in which the body's own tissues are attacked by the immune system. These treatments' capacity to modulate the immune system has the potential to revolutionize medicine by providing fresh methods for treating complicated illnesses. Immunotherapies may eventually become a crucial part of treating a wide range of illnesses beyond cancer as a result of this diversification.

Artificial Intelligence's Function:

The future of immunotherapy is anticipated to be significantly influenced by artificial intelligence (AI). Large volumes of patient data, including genetic profiles and treatment outcomes, can be analyzed by AI systems. They can help clinicians make better informed treatment decisions by doing this. AI may be used to optimize treatment regimens for improved patient outcomes, identify possible adverse effects early, and forecast which individuals are most likely to respond to particular immunotherapies. AI in healthcare has the potential to completely transform the medical field and improve the accuracy of treatment choices.

Worldwide Availability and Cost Effectiveness:

We will continue to be dedicated to improving immunotherapy's affordability and accessibility on a global scale. There are existing programs and joint efforts in place to lower the cost of these therapies, promote international collaboration, and guarantee that all patients, regardless of where they live or how much money they have, get fair access to these life-changing treatments. In addition to advancing scientific understanding, the future of immunotherapy lies in making sure that the advantages of these breakthroughs are distributed globally.

As we look to the future of immunotherapy, we see a highly personalized medical environment where each patient's profile is precisely catered to. Immunotherapy is positioned to be at the vanguard of this fascinating scientific journey, providing new hope and opportunities for patients worldwide. The arsenal against cancer and numerous diseases is growing quickly.

CHAPTER 13
The Effects of Immunotherapy Outside of Medicine

Immunotherapy has a profound impact on many facets of society, including patient advocacy and economics, even outside the field of medicine. This chapter explores the wider implications of immunotherapy, emphasizing how it affects various facets of life.

Economic Consequences:

The use of immunotherapy has spurred a new economic revolution. The biotechnology and pharmaceutical industries have seen large financial investments and employment growth as a result of the discovery and commercialization of immunotherapies. The high price of various immunotherapies has also sparked questions about affordability and the long-term viability of healthcare budgets.

Patient Empowerment and Advocacy:

Patients can now actively participate in their own care because to immunotherapy. In order to advance treatment equity, increase awareness, and advance research, patients and advocacy groups are speaking out more and more. Their combined efforts have sparked improvements in funding for research, legislation, and patient and family assistance.

The Impact on Innovation and Research:

Novel immunotherapies such as Keytruda have completely changed the field of cancer research. Researchers and organizations are devoting more time and funds to learning about the immune system's connections to cancer. Research on immunotherapy is having an impact on various areas of medicine, with the potential to provide novel treatments for illnesses other than cancer.

Shifting the Paradigm of Treatment:

Conventional therapeutic paradigms have been questioned by immunotherapy. The efficacy of immunotherapies in treating specific tumors has led to a reassessment of treatment protocols and tactics. Immunotherapy is currently a front-line option in some cancer regimens, establishing it as a key player in the fight against the illness.

Working Together Internationally:

International cooperation has been required for the development and implementation of immunotherapies. Global collaboration among researchers, medical experts, and regulatory bodies is fostering knowledge exchange, developing treatment protocols, and guaranteeing that these innovative treatments are accessible to all.

Social and Ethical Aspects to Consider:

Ethical concerns around benefit distribution, price, and accessibility are brought up by immunotherapy. Society will need to address concerns about resource allocation and equal access as these treatments advance. Moreover, when immunotherapies become more widely used outside of the cancer field, ethical debates over the use of human immune system enhancement for the prevention or treatment of other diseases may arise.

Educative Repercussions:

In the field of education, immunotherapy has an impact. The most recent developments in immunotherapy are being incorporated into medical and healthcare curricula, guaranteeing that medical practitioners are equipped to administer these therapies. Initiatives for patient education are also being developed to enhance comprehension and promote well-informed decision-making.

Public Knowledge and the Mass Media:

The public's awareness is growing and headlines featuring immunotherapy success stories are becoming more frequent. In addition to demystifying complicated medical concepts and giving patients and their families hope and inspiration, the media is a vital source of information about these treatments.

The Path Forward:

The application of immunotherapy outside of medicine is still developing. The impact of immunotherapy on our lives is probably going to increase as science progresses, the economy changes, and social norms adjust. These therapies' future place in healthcare and society will be greatly influenced by the larger conversation that surrounds them, particularly with regard to their accessibility and affordability.

An overview of the complex consequences of immunotherapy on different aspects of our lives is given in this chapter. Immunotherapy's lasting impact is demonstrated by the changes it has made to the domains of healthcare, economy, and society.

Economic Consequences:

The development of immunotherapy has had a big impact on the economy. The biotechnology and pharmaceutical industries have made significant financial expenditures in the research, testing, and commercialization of immunotherapies. High-paying positions in industry, research and development, and healthcare delivery have resulted from this. In many places, the biotech industry's rapid growth is a major factor in economic expansion.

Concurrently, questions concerning the sustainability and affordability of healthcare have been highlighted by the high expense of certain immunotherapies, especially when they are administered for lengthy periods of time. Talks on medicine access, insurance coverage, and pricing structures have become necessary as a result of this economic crisis. For healthcare systems around the world, striking a balance between innovation and cost-effectiveness continues to be a major problem.

Patient Empowerment and Advocacy:

Patients now have the ability to actively participate in their healthcare journey because to immunotherapy. Patient advocacy groups have played a crucial role in advancing research, increasing public awareness, and promoting fair access to therapies. These groups are led by people who have personally experienced the life-changing effects of immunotherapy. Patient and family assistance has improved, research funding has increased, and policies have changed as a result of the collective voice of patients.

Thanks to the abundance of information available to them, patients may now make well-informed judgments on their treatment options when it comes to immunotherapy. People are playing a bigger part in determining the direction of medicine in the age of patient-centric care.

The Impact on Innovation and Research:

The advent of immunotherapies such as Keytruda has revolutionized the field of cancer research. Researching the immune system and how it interacts with cancer cells is a major focus for scientists. Research on immunotherapy is not just affecting oncology; it is also having an impact on other areas of medicine.

Innovations in fields like gene therapy, which uses the immune system to treat illnesses other than cancer, have been sparked by research into immunotherapy. The collaboration of many fields is paving the way for immunotherapy to become a major component of medical innovation in the future, providing fresh methods for treating a variety of diseases.

Shifting the Paradigm of Treatment:

The conventional paradigms of cancer treatment have been called into question by immunotherapy. Reevaluating treatment sequences and tactics has become necessary due to the efficacy of immunotherapies in certain forms of cancer. Immunotherapy is currently used as a first-line treatment for some malignancies, making it a key element in the fight against the illness. Long-term survival rates and patient outcomes may be enhanced by this paradigm change.

Working Together Internationally:

Collaboration between nations is necessary for the development and implementation of immunotherapies. Global collaboration among researchers, medical experts, and regulatory bodies is fostering knowledge exchange, developing treatment protocols, and guaranteeing that these innovative treatments are accessible to all. International cooperation promotes the sharing of best practices, clinical data, and ideas, improving patient outcomes everywhere.

Social and Ethical Aspects to Consider:

There are significant ethical questions raised by immunotherapy. As the area develops, equal access, cost, and resource allocation will become more pressing social challenges. To guarantee that the benefits of immunotherapy are distributed fairly, ethical issues pertaining to benefit distribution and the abolition of treatment access inequities must be resolved.

Immunotherapies may spark moral debates concerning the use of human immune system enhancement for the prevention or treatment of other diseases as they become more widely used beyond cancer. The proper use of potent biotechnologies and the possible societal repercussions of immune system changes will be the main topics of debate throughout these sessions.

Educative Repercussions:

Immunotherapy has a noticeable impact on education as well. The most recent developments in immunotherapy are being incorporated into medical and healthcare curriculum, ensuring that medical personnel are equipped to provide these cutting-edge treatments. The aforementioned educational modifications equip healthcare practitioners with the essential competencies and understanding to make well-informed treatment decisions, efficiently monitor patients, and effectively handle potential adverse effects.

Furthermore, educational programs are being created to help patients better comprehend immunotherapy. This include giving patients and their families educational materials, information in plain language, and techniques for making well-informed decisions about available treatment alternatives. Patient education programs are designed to provide people the knowledge and skills they need to actively participate in their healthcare decisions and make educated treatment decisions.

Public Knowledge and the Mass Media:

The media has begun to focus more on immunotherapy, featuring success stories on a regular basis. In addition to demystifying complicated medical concepts and giving patients and their families hope and inspiration, the media is a vital source of information about these treatments. The public's knowledge and comprehension of immunotherapy are further enhanced by the treatment's growing prominence in the media.

In addition to raising awareness of the possible advantages of immunotherapy, public awareness also encourages advocacy, financing for research, and improved patient-provider interaction. When people are diagnosed with cancer and learn that there are cutting-edge treatments like immunotherapy, it gives them hope and optimism.

The Path Forward:

The impact of immunotherapy outside of medicine is still developing. The influence of immunotherapy is projected to increase with further study, shifting economic ramifications, and adapting societal issues. These treatments' future place in healthcare and society will be greatly influenced by the larger conversation that surrounds them, particularly with regard to their accessibility and affordability.

In conclusion, immunotherapy has an impact on many aspects of our life and goes well beyond the field of medicine. The changes brought about by immunotherapy

CHAPTER 14
Immunotherapy's Boundaries and Ethical Dilemmas

Given its amazing potential to revolutionize the way cancer and other diseases are treated, immunotherapy raises a number of moral questions that need to be carefully considered. The complicated ethical environment surrounding immunotherapy and its limitations is examined in this chapter.

Equity in Patient Selection:

The fair patient selection process is one of the main moral conundrums in immunotherapy. It can be difficult to determine which patients will benefit the most because not all patients respond in the same way. This raises concerns about how scarce resources are allocated and the possibility of unequal access to therapies that can save lives. To guarantee that choices regarding patient selection are made in an equitable and open manner, ethical frameworks and rules are required.

Accessibility and Affordability:

Due to the high price of various immunotherapies, questions of accessibility and affordability have been raised. It is morally required to guarantee that all patients, regardless of their financial situation, have access to these cutting-edge medicines. It is a difficult ethical task to strike a balance between the necessity for pharmaceutical corporations to recover their expenditures associated with research and development and giving patients inexpensive access.

Autonomy of the Patient and Informed Consent:

Clinical trials and innovative medicines are frequently a part of immunotherapy. It can be particularly difficult to provide informed consent in this situation, because patients fully grasp the potential risks and advantages. It is ethical to make sure patients are informed about the intricacies of immunotherapy and given the freedom to choose how they want to be treated.

Genomics and Privacy:

It could be necessary to gather and examine a lot of patient genetic and medical data in order to administer immunotherapy. It is necessary to address ethical concerns about data security, privacy, and the possible exploitation of genetic information. It is a difficult ethical task to strike a balance between expanding medical knowledge and protecting patients' private information.

Getting Past Resistance:

Ethical questions are also raised by the creation of methods to combat immunotherapy resistance. These strategies, which might make use of innovative interventions or adaptive therapies, need to be carefully considered in light of patient safety and well-being.

Boosting Immunity in Humans:

Ethical debates regarding boosting the human immune system to prevent or treat a range of ailments may surface as immunotherapy's potential uses extend beyond the treatment of disease. This starts a conversation regarding the moral applications of biotechnologies and the effects on society of altering the immune system for different goals.

Ethics in Clinical Trials:

The area of immunotherapy must advance through clinical trials. But there are ethical questions about how these trials are planned, carried out, and reported. Crucial ethical concerns include making sure that trial participants receive the finest treatment possible, are treated with the highest respect, and that trial results are openly and truthfully communicated.

International Cooperation and Access:

119

International cooperation is necessary to guarantee universal access to immunotherapy and benefit sharing. Addressing inequities in treatment access and the prudent administration of resources and benefits globally are examples of ethical considerations.

Public Education and Awareness:

It is crucial to educate people about immunotherapy and engage in ethical communication. Ethical difficulties that need to be addressed include making sure patients completely understand their treatment options, encouraging awareness without setting unreasonable expectations, and responsibly disseminating information in plain language.

The Path Forward:

Immunotherapy's ethical conundrums require constant navigation. Due to the complexity of these issues, a multidisciplinary strategy involving physicians, ethicists, legislators, patients, and the general public is required. To make sure that the potential of immunotherapy is used responsibly and ethically, it will be essential to set precise ethical norms and have lively conversations on these subjects. The ethical issues surrounding immunotherapy will become more and more important as the field develops and shapes its future.

Equity in Patient Selection:

Selecting the patients who will most benefit from immunotherapy is a difficult and morally delicate decision. Even while these therapies have shown a great deal of effectiveness, not everyone responds to them. This begs the dilemma of how to fairly choose patients so that those who could benefit can receive treatment without going overboard with those who might not respond favorably. These choices must be made in accordance with ethical frameworks in order to guarantee that patient selection is open, supported by data, and centered on providing the greatest results for specific people.

Accessibility and Affordability:

One controversial ethical issue with certain immunotherapies is their high cost. It is a difficult task to strike a balance between the requirement that pharmaceutical companies recover their research and development costs and the need to make these treatments accessible and cheap for all patients. It makes people talk about insurance policies, cost structures, and the role that governments and healthcare systems play in making sure that the wealthy are not the only ones who can access life-saving therapies.

Autonomy of the Patient and Informed Consent:

Clinical studies, novel therapies, and intricate medical knowledge are frequently associated with immunotherapy. This calls into question patient autonomy and informed consent in an ethical manner. Patients need to be completely aware of the advantages and disadvantages of their course of treatment, as well as the fact that certain procedures are experimental. Even in the case of novel and untested treatments, they ought to be granted the freedom to choose how they want to be treated. Healthcare professionals have an ethical duty to ensure sure patients are able to make educated decisions while navigating the complexities of immunotherapy.

Genomics and Privacy:

Genetic and medical information from patients is often used by immunotherapy to customize treatment. This raises moral questions about data security, privacy, and the appropriate management of private genetic data. Encouraging medical research while maintaining patient privacy requires careful ethical balancing. To guarantee that patient genetic and medical data is utilized responsibly, strong data protection protocols, openness, and adherence to ethical norms are necessary.

Getting Past Resistance:

There are moral dilemmas in the development of methods to combat immunotherapy resistance. These strategies could make use of cutting-edge interventions or adaptive therapy. Ethical issues encompass patient welfare, safety, and a meticulous assessment of the advantages and disadvantages of these treatments. A primary priority is striking a balance between the likelihood of therapy success and the well-being of patients.

Boosting Immunity in Humans:

The application of immunotherapy to conditions other than disease treatment raises moral questions regarding boosting the human immune system. Despite the enormous potential advantages, there are ethical issues to be addressed, such as the appropriate application of biotechnologies and the social ramifications of altering the immune system for objectives other than preserving health.

Ethics in Clinical Trials:

Immunotherapy advancement depends on clinical trials, however there are ethical issues with them. It is morally required to make sure that, even in a trial context, participants are respected and receive the greatest treatment possible. Furthermore, scientific advancement and safeguarding the interests of trial participants and the larger patient community depend heavily on openness and accuracy in publishing trial outcomes.

International Cooperation and Access:

International cooperation is necessary to provide fair access to and benefit sharing from immunotherapy. Addressing inequities in treatment access and the prudent administration of resources and benefits globally are examples of ethical considerations. One of the main ethical challenges is making sure that immunotherapy reaches patients in underprivileged areas and that the benefits are shared equally.

Public Education and Awareness:

It is crucial to communicate and educate about immunotherapy in an ethical manner. It entails raising awareness without instilling irrational expectations, properly distributing information about these treatments, and simplifying difficult medical terms. Ensuring the public and patients have access to information that is truthful, moral, and impartial is essential to fostering educated decision-making and protecting patient autonomy.

Addressing these difficult moral conundrums will be essential as immunotherapy develops in order to guarantee that its promise is used sensibly and morally. The future of immunotherapy will be shaped in large part by interdisciplinary conversations involving medical professionals, ethicists, legislators, patients, and the general public in a way that upholds the ethical precepts of justice, autonomy, beneficence, and non-maleficence.

CHAPTER 15
Immunotherapy Ethics's Future

The ethical issues surrounding immunotherapy will change concurrently with its ongoing revolution in medicine. This chapter explores the new ethical advances and difficulties that are arising in the field of immunotherapy.

Ethical Precision and Personalized Medicine:

Immunotherapy is set to grow much more specialized and accurate in the future. Navigating this terrain and ensuring that patients receive treatments specific to their individual genetic and immunological profiles will be the main ethical concerns. The development of increasingly precise treatments will continue to be guided by the ethical ideal of beneficence, which is doing what is best for the patient.

Access and Equity in Healthcare:

Ensuring fair access to these cutting-edge medicines will continue to be a primary ethical challenge as immunotherapy develops. Regardless of a patient's socioeconomic background or geographic location, the goal of making immunotherapy available to all will be guided by the idea of justice, which promotes fairness and equal distribution of benefits.

Security and Privacy of Data:

Data security and privacy will become even more of an ethical concern in the future when medical and genetic data are used to determine treatment options. In order to guarantee patient data security, ethical frameworks must address the appropriate management of sensitive patient information, placing a strong emphasis on openness, consent, and data protection procedures.

Algorithms and Ethics in AI:

Ethical issues will arise when artificial intelligence (AI) is used in healthcare, particularly immunotherapy. Treatment choices will be guided by AI-driven algorithms, and the moral use of AI in clinical settings will gain attention. AI will be developed and implemented in accordance with ethical standards to guarantee that patient autonomy is respected and that patient care is improved.

New Emerging Ethical Conundrums:

The development of immunotherapy will give rise to new moral conundrums. These could involve concerns regarding the moral application of biotechnologies for both medical and non-medical uses, as well as how to strengthen the human immune system beyond the treatment of sickness. Under the guiding concepts of beneficence, non-maleficence, and autonomy, ethical discourse will address these intricate problems.

International Cooperation and Ethical Alliances:

International cooperation will be essential to immunotherapy's future. The appropriate management of resources, benefit sharing, and multinational relationships will all be subject to ethical considerations. The tenets of beneficence and justice will direct initiatives to guarantee that immunotherapy reaches patients everywhere, promoting fair access and benefit sharing.

The Public's Awareness and Ethical Education:

Public awareness and ethical education will be given more weight in the ethics of immunotherapy in the future. To make educated judgments, patients, healthcare providers, and the general public will require access to ethical knowledge and tools. Respect for autonomy as an ethical concept will highlight the significance of informed consent and patient-centered care.

Ethical Supervision and Law:

The need for ethical supervision and control will grow as immunotherapy progresses. In order to guarantee that ethical standards are respected in clinical trials, therapy, and research, regulatory agencies and groups will be crucial. Data privacy, fair access to therapies, and patient safety will all be under this watchful eye.

Balance of Ethics in Advancements:

It will always be difficult to strike a balance between ethical issues and the growth of science and medicine. The responsible development and application of immunotherapy will be guided by ethical standards. The future of immunotherapy will revolve around achieving a balanced balance between advancement and moral considerations.

The field of immunotherapy ethics is in a state of constant flux, influenced by social shifts, continuing scientific discoveries, and developing moral principles. Immunotherapy is a ground-breaking discipline that promises to benefit patients indefinitely while maintaining the highest ethical standards. Responsibility and patient-centered development in this sector will be predicated on ethical principles.

Ethical Precision and Personalized Medicine:

Immunotherapy may lead to even more individualized and accurate therapies in the future. Advances in immune system profiling and genetics will allow treatments to be customized to the unique features of each patient's malignancy. The ethical principle of beneficence, which emphasizes acting in the patient's best interest, is in line with this individualized approach. But this level of accuracy also brings with it complex ethical issues. It becomes essential to strike a balance between offering the best possible care and making sure that it is within everyone's means. Ethical frameworks will have to deal with things like equitable distribution of these incredibly customized medicines and how to handle situations in which the most exact treatment might not be available or appropriate for some people.

Access and Equity in Healthcare:

As immunotherapy develops, access to healthcare equity will remain a major ethical challenge. Fairness and an equal distribution of rewards are important, and this is emphasized by the justice principle. It is crucial to guarantee that patients, irrespective of their geographic location or socioeconomic level, have access to state-of-the-art immunotherapies. Innovative approaches are required to address this ethical dilemma, such as global collaboration, cost-cutting strategies, and tenacious patient advocacy to overcome inequalities in healthcare results and access.

Security and Privacy of Data:

Data security and privacy will become more important ethical concerns as immunotherapy uses more genetic and medical data. It is morally required to protect private medical data. It will be necessary for ethical frameworks to address responsible patient data handling. Patients' trust and confidence will be crucially maintained by ensuring transparency in the use of data, gaining informed consent for data collection, and putting strict data protection measures in place.

Algorithms and Ethics in AI:

There are ethical concerns with the use of artificial intelligence (AI) in healthcare, particularly with the creation of algorithms that direct treatment choices. The proper application of AI to improve patient care will be the main ethical focus. It is crucial to make sure AI upholds the values of beneficence, non-maleficence (doing no harm), and patient autonomy. Guidelines for preventing prejudice and discrimination in AI-driven healthcare decisions as well as ensuring that AI enhances rather than compromises patient well-being will be part of ethical oversight.

135

New Emerging Ethical Conundrums:

As immunotherapy develops, new moral conundrums will arise, such as the possibility of using immune system enhancement for objectives other than the cure of disease. The proper application of biotechnologies and their social ramifications will be central to ethical discourse. The ethical concepts of beneficence (maximizing benefits), non-maleficence (minimizing harm), and autonomy (respect for human choices) will serve as the framework for these talks. These moral discussions will support the development of science and technology and help direct its responsible applications.

International Cooperation and Ethical Alliances:

Immunotherapy will require more international cooperation in the future to guarantee benefit sharing and fair access. The appropriate management of resources, benefit sharing, and multinational relationships will all be subject to ethical considerations. The tenets of beneficence and justice will direct initiatives to guarantee that immunotherapy reaches patients everywhere, promoting fair access and benefit sharing. These worldwide cooperation will be shaped and their commitment to ethical standards ensured by the implementation of ethical frameworks.

The Public's Awareness and Ethical Education:

The significance of public awareness and ethical education will grow in the future. To make educated judgments, patients, healthcare providers, and the general public will require access to ethical knowledge and tools. Respect for autonomy, an ethical ideal that emphasizes the value of informed consent, patient-centered care, and moral treatment decisions, will be crucial. Encouraging a knowledgeable, conscious, and morally involved public is essential to guaranteeing that patients actively participate in the process of making healthcare decisions.

Ethical Supervision and Law:

The need for ethical supervision and control of immunotherapy will only grow. In order to guarantee that ethical standards are respected in clinical trials, therapy, and research, regulatory agencies and groups will be crucial. Ethical supervision will cover topics including fair access to therapies, patient safety, and data protection. It is imperative to uphold ethical norms in the advancement and implementation of immunotherapy to safeguard patient welfare and preserve public confidence.

Balance of Ethics in Advancements:

It will always be difficult to strike a balance between ethical issues and the growth of science and medicine. The appropriate development and application of immunotherapy will be guided by the constantly changing ethical landscape, which functions as a compass. The future of immunotherapy will revolve around finding a balance between advancement and moral obligations, making sure that this novel field maintains the greatest moral standards while continuing to help patients. As immunotherapy develops, morality will be essential to responsible, patient-centered advances in healthcare, reinforcing the dedication to moral and just healthcare provision.

CHAPTER 16
Immunotherapy's Effects on Society and Culture

Beyond the acute medical consequences, immunotherapy has a significant and far-reaching impact on society and culture. The impact of immunotherapy on society and culture is examined in this chapter.

Taking on the Stigma of Cancer:

The effectiveness of immunotherapy in treating cancer dispels common myths and stigmas associated with the illness. Immunotherapy helps alter the way society views and discusses cancer by offering hope and improved treatment outcomes. By sharing their experiences and changing the narrative from one of dread to one of resiliency and hope, patients and survivors take on the role of advocates.

Changing the Treatment Paradigm:

Immunotherapy has changed the way that cancer is treated. It provides a more focused, non-intrusive, and possibly more successful method. This change affects society's expectations for healthcare as well as the experiences of cancer patients. Immunotherapy is changing how we approach treatment throughout the medical spectrum as it becomes available for more disorders.

Giving Patients Power:

Immunotherapy gives patients the ability to take a more active and knowledgeable role in their own care. The focus on collaborative decision-making and individualized medicine puts patients at the center of their treatment regimens. Patients are more actively involved in influencing healthcare decisions and discussions because they are knowledgeable participants in their treatment.

Innovation in Technology and Medicine:

Immunotherapy's success is an example of the best kind of medical and technological innovation. The amazing progress made in the treatment of life-threatening diseases is celebrated by society, which is motivated by the transformational potential of science. Support for scientific research and heightened public interest in healthcare are frequent examples of this inspiration.

Implications for Policy and the Economy:

Immunotherapy has consequences for policy and the economy outside of the medical domain. These treatments are quite expensive, which raises questions regarding access, insurance, and healthcare budgets. Economists and policymakers struggle to find a balance between affordability and innovation, which has an impact on how resources are distributed in the healthcare industry.

Global Equity and Health:

Immunotherapy draws attention to the discrepancies in global health and the value of universal access to healthcare. It emphasizes how crucial it is for nations to work together in order to guarantee that cutting-edge medical treatments are accessible to everyone. The impact on society is an increased consciousness of global health concerns and the need for the allocation of healthcare resources in an ethical manner.

Inspirational Stories and Cultural Narratives:

Immunotherapy produces uplifting tales of tenacity and survival. These stories are found in many literary works, motion pictures, and social media platforms. Stories of people using immunotherapy to overcome illnesses like cancer and other conditions have the power to influence societal narratives about bravery, hope, and advancements in medicine.

Knowledge and Consciousness:

Immunotherapy promotes understanding of intricate medical ideas and has a significant educational influence. It inspires people to look for a better comprehension of science, genetics, and healthcare. A society that is more knowledgeable and health-conscious may result from this educational transition.

Obstacles to Social and Ethical Standards:

Immunotherapy challenges ethical and societal conventions while pushing the limits of treatment. It is important to carefully analyze the societal and cultural ramifications of discussions surrounding the ethical use of biotechnologies and the augmentation of the human immune system.

The Function of Communication and the Media:

The media is essential for spreading knowledge about immunotherapy. It influences how the general public views and is aware of medical breakthroughs. For society to promote correct understanding and well-informed discussions, media reporting must be ethical and responsible.

Immunotherapy has a wide range of social and cultural effects, including viewpoint changes, patient empowerment, and motivational stories of recovery from disease. Immunotherapy will have a profoundly different impact on how we view science, medicine, and human nature as it develops. It emphasizes how scientific advancement and cultural change interact dynamically.

Taking on the Stigma of Cancer:

The effectiveness of immunotherapy in treating cancer has played a significant role in challenging and destroying prevailing stigmas and misconceptions about the illness. For individuals who have been diagnosed with cancer, it offers a glimmer of hope despite being viewed as a fearsome foe. The conventional narrative of cancer as an unavoidable death sentence is challenged by the transforming potential of immunotherapy, which substitutes it with one of resiliency, hope, and the prospect of a future. After receiving immunotherapy, some patients go on to become activists, sharing their experiences and helping to alter public opinion. Instead of facing cancer with dread and despair, they encourage others to do so with courage and optimism.

Changing the Treatment Paradigm:

The paradigm of cancer treatment has significantly changed with the advent of immunotherapy. When compared to more conventional treatments like radiation and chemotherapy, it provides a more focused, minimally intrusive, and maybe more successful method. This change not only improves the quality of life for cancer patients but also modifies society's expectations for medical care. Immunotherapy is challenging long-standing healthcare norms and paradigms as it develops and spreads to treat diseases other than cancer. This has prompted a more comprehensive reevaluation of how we approach and comprehend treatment throughout the medical spectrum.

Giving Patients Power:

Immunotherapy gives patients more control over their healthcare by putting them front and center. Patients are encouraged to participate more actively in their treatment plans and become better informed by the emphasis on shared decision-making and individualized therapy. Patients actively participate in determining the course of their healthcare journey in conjunction with their healthcare providers. Not only does this patient-centric approach produce better results, but it also empowers people to take greater responsibility for their health and cultivates a deeper sense of autonomy and empowerment.

Innovation in Technology and Medicine:

147

The best of medical and technical innovation is reflected in the success of immunotherapy. It enthralls society by demonstrating the revolutionary potential of science. The immunotherapy advances are a source of inspiration and gratitude for the technological and scientific advances in medicine. The public is interested in science and healthcare because of the amazing progress made in using the immune system to fight disease. This motivation frequently results in more funding for scientific research, promoting a society that values creativity and ground-breaking discoveries.

Implications for Policy and the Economy:

There have been many arguments regarding the economic and policy implications of healthcare due to the high cost of certain immunotherapies. Economists and policymakers struggle to strike a balance between affordability and innovation. These talks push the limits of ethics and policy, affecting how resources are allocated in the healthcare industry. It becomes a question of social justice and healthcare ethics to figure out how to provide fair access to these ground-breaking treatments, highlighting the need to address the legislative and financial components of healthcare access.

Global Equity and Health:

Immunotherapy draws attention to the essential need for fair access to healthcare and the gaps in global health. It examines differences in healthcare access between regions and populations and highlights the idea that everyone has the right to good health. This has had an impact on society by raising awareness of global health challenges and advocating for the ethical distribution of healthcare resources. It encourages worldwide cooperation in the pursuit of global health equity and cultivates a feeling of shared accountability for addressing healthcare disparities.

Inspirational Stories and Cultural Narratives:

Immunotherapy produces uplifting tales of survival and resiliency that seep into society. Books, movies, social media, and other cultural forms of expression all incorporate these stories. They have the power to influence larger cultural narratives by fostering courage, hope, and confidence in the advancement of medicine. Inspirational tales of people using immunotherapy to beat cancer and other illnesses frequently become into icons of overcoming adversity and shape societal perceptions of the resiliency of the human spirit.

Knowledge and Consciousness:

Immunotherapy promotes increased public knowledge and understanding of intricate medical ideas, such as the immune system's function in the management of cancer. The public is encouraged to pursue a better understanding of healthcare, genetics, and scientific innovation by the success stories and the supporting science. A more knowledgeable and health-conscious society that recognizes the worth of scientific research, the complexity of medical treatments, and the significance of taking preventative measures for one's health and well-being may result from this shift in educational approach.

Obstacles to Social and Ethical Standards:

Immunotherapy challenges accepted social standards and ethical bounds as it advances the frontiers of treatment. Questions of ethics and culture come up when we talk about boosting the human immune system, possibly for uses other than curing illness. Navigating these intricate difficulties will need society to think carefully about how to use biotechnologies responsibly and what social ramifications might result from immune system alterations. The maximizing of benefits (beneficence), the mitigation of harm (non-maleficence), and respect for personal autonomy will all be guiding concepts in these debates.

The Function of Communication and the Media:

The public's opinion of immunotherapy is greatly influenced by the media. The media's ethical and responsible reporting is crucial to promoting truthful perceptions and well-informed conversations in society. Cultural narratives and public understanding are shaped by how the media presents the advantages, difficulties, and moral dilemmas associated with immunotherapy. Building an informed and morally engaged public requires ethical and knowledgeable communication in the media. The media's power to shape public opinion emphasizes the relationship between advancements in science and cultural change.

Immunotherapy has a wide range of social and cultural effects, including viewpoint changes, patient empowerment, and motivational stories of recovery from disease. Immunotherapy will have a profoundly different impact on how we view science, medicine, and human nature as it develops. It highlights the dynamic interaction between scientific advancement and cultural change, demonstrating how developments in medicine have the power to uplift society and influence cultural narratives.

CHAPTER 17
Immunotherapy's Future and Uncharted Territories

Immunotherapy's future is an exciting voyage into unexplored territory where science, technology, and medicine come together to solve cutting-edge problems and open up fresh opportunities. We investigate the unknown areas that lay ahead in this chapter.

New Therapeutic Pathways:

Immunotherapy's future has the prospect of revealing numerous uncharted therapeutic territories. Immunotherapy will become more widely used to treat a greater variety of illnesses in addition to its present efficacy in treating cancer. Novel immunotherapeutic techniques may be used to treat infectious infections, degenerative ailments, and autoimmune disorders. This extension will completely change the way we think about illnesses that have long eluded a viable cure.

Synergistic methods and combination therapies:

Future developments will see combination medicines assume a central role. Researchers are looking into the ways in which immunotherapy can work in concert with other medical interventions, including as conventional medicines like radiation and chemotherapy, to provide even more potent and successful results. Optimizing these combinations to minimize adverse effects and guarantee the best possible patient care is the difficult part.

Improving Customization

Immunotherapy will become even more customized in the future. Plans for therapy will be guided by developments in immunological profiling, genetics, and the understanding of individual variances. With the advancement of precision medicine, patients will receive precisely customized medicines based on their own genetic and immunological composition. The cornerstone of healthcare going forward will be personalized immunotherapy, which maximizes benefits and reduces side effects.

Reaching Past Cancer:

Even while immunotherapy has already revolutionized the field of cancer treatment, its applications will only grow. Treatments for neurological disorders, viral diseases, and autoimmune disorders will be among the new paths that may provide a better way to treat or even cure problems that were thought to be incurable.

The Moral Dilemmas of Improvement:

Ethical concerns will surface when immunotherapy's potential goes beyond curing illness to include boosting the immune system for other goals. The idea of bio-enhancement for purposes other than medicine will go against ethical and societal conventions. The main topics of discussion will be safety, equity, and the moral application of biotechnologies to alter human nature.

Predictive medicine and AI:

The use of artificial intelligence (AI) in immunotherapy will be significant in the future. To forecast how a patient will respond to treatment, spot possible adverse effects, and improve treatments, machine learning algorithms will be employed. When AI is used to make important medical choices, ethical issues such as responsibility, openness, and responsible data use will come into play.

International Cooperation for All-Access:

To guarantee that immunotherapy's benefits are distributed worldwide, increased international cooperation will be necessary. Efforts to ensure universal access to these innovative medications and address global health inequities will be guided by the ethical principles of beneficence and fairness. To achieve equal access, cooperation between governments, groups, and pharmaceutical firms will be essential.

Instruction and Public Participation:

It will be essential to educate the public and medical professionals in the uncertain future of immunotherapy. To make sure that people are informed of their treatment options, the ethical issues surrounding these medicines, and the necessity of making responsible decisions, public participation will be promoted. Education programs will help close the knowledge gap between science and society, resulting in more knowledgeable and capable people.

Regulation and Policy:

Strong laws and restrictions will be needed for immunotherapy in the future. The observance of ethical norms in clinical trials, therapy, and research will be guaranteed by these recommendations. The role of organizations and regulatory authorities in ensuring patient safety and data security will grow in importance as immunotherapy becomes more widespread.

Handling Unexpected Obstacles:

Unexpected obstacles abound in unexplored territory. Unexpected hazards may call for cautious attention, and new findings may present moral conundrums. Immunotherapy's future will require adaptability, flexibility, and responsible reactions to new problems.

The unexplored areas of immunotherapy present countless opportunities as well as fresh ethical dilemmas. Ethical concepts will always be at the center of responsible, patient-centered technological and scientific advancements. Immunotherapy is an exciting new field that society has to explore with an ethical compass to make sure the amazing benefits of these treatments are used sensibly and fairly.

New Therapeutic Pathways:

Immunotherapy's future is about to reveal a wealth of uncharted treatment territories. Even if the field's effectiveness in treating cancer is already astounding, scientists are excited to explore new ground. Among these is the potential for immunotherapy to completely transform the treatment of autoimmune diseases, which was traditionally believed to be outside the purview of contemporary medicine. The possibility of reprogramming the immune system to fight infectious diseases, such as HIV and newly developing viruses, is an uncharted territory. Furthermore, the use of immunotherapy in neurodegenerative disorders makes therapies and interventions possible that have the potential to significantly improve the lives of millions of people with illnesses like Parkinson's and Alzheimer's. The ethical questions around these therapies' responsible and fair use are growing along with them.

Synergistic methods and combination therapies:

Combination medicines will become a formidable force in the undiscovered future. By attempting to maximize immunotherapy's potential through synergistic techniques, scientists are making groundbreaking discoveries. It might be difficult to balance immunotherapy with more conventional treatments like radiation and chemotherapy. The main goal of this endeavor is to maximize therapy effectiveness while avoiding negative effects. Ensuring that these combinations are designed with patient well-being as the primary priority and that their deployment complies with beneficence and non-maleficence principles will be the focus of ethical considerations.

Improving Customization

Treatment plan customisation will advance to previously unheard-of levels in the future. Precision medicine will be shaped by developments in genomics, immunological profiling, and our comprehension of individual genetic differences. The course of treatment will be personalized for each patient based on their distinct genetic and immunological profile. This development highlights the moral significance of optimizing benefits and reducing damage and captures the spirit of individualized treatment. Ethical standards require that these customized therapies be available and reasonably priced, guaranteeing that each patient has an equal chance to gain.

Reaching Past Cancer:

Immunotherapy has already taken the cancer treatment world by storm, but there is still more unexplored territory for it to explore. There may be new hope for diseases that were previously thought to be incurable. Immunotherapy can help autoimmune diseases like lupus and multiple sclerosis by reducing the overactivity of the immune system. Immunotherapeutic remedies to infectious diseases such as HIV, for which a cure has proven difficult, may be attainable. New treatments for neurological diseases like ALS and Alzheimer's may be able to stop or even reverse their terrible progression. The frontiers of healthcare will be reinterpreted as a result of this growth into new fields, opening up new avenues for medical advancement.

The Moral Dilemmas of Improvement:

The distinction between improving an immune system and treating a disease is becoming more hazy as immunotherapy develops. The idea of boosting the immune system of humans for non-medical reasons defies ethical and social conventions. Safety, equality, and the right application of biotechnologies to transform humankind are all matters of ethical concern. As we venture into new territory, discussions will include subjects like immune system improvement for lifespan, performance, and resilience, pushing the limits of ethical reasoning.

Predictive medicine and AI:

In the future, immunotherapy will require the use of artificial intelligence (AI). Algorithms utilizing machine learning techniques will forecast treatment outcomes, detect possible adverse reactions, and enhance treatment plans. Transparency, accountability, and the prudent use of patient data are necessary for the ethical application of AI in making crucial medical choices. In order to make sure that AI in medicine adheres to the values of beneficence and patient autonomy, it must be carefully supervised ethically.

International Cooperation for All-Access:

To guarantee that immunotherapy's benefits are distributed worldwide, increased international cooperation will be necessary. Encouraging universal access to these innovative cures and resolving global health inequities will be made possible by the ethical principles of beneficence and justice. This calls for cooperation between countries as well as between pharmaceutical corporations and international organizations. It emphasizes the moral duty to see to it that patients everywhere have equitable access to care.

Instruction and Public Participation:

In the uncertain realm of immunotherapy, public involvement and education will be essential. This will create a bridge between society and science, empowering and enlightening people. It is essential that the general public understands complicated medical terms and the moral issues related to these treatments. Enabling people to make knowledgeable decisions regarding their health will be essential to the ethical development of immunotherapy.

Regulation and Policy:

Strong laws and rules must be created in the future of immunotherapy to guarantee the upholding of moral principles. Immunotherapy is expanding into new sectors of healthcare, and protecting patient safety and data security will require ethical monitoring. The creation and application of these ground-breaking treatments will present an ethical dilemma: how to innovate while maintaining patient safety.

Handling Unexpected Obstacles:

Uncharted ground is by its very nature uncertain. Unexpected difficulties will surely surface as science and technology advance. Unexpected risks may require careful attention, and new discoveries may present ethical conundrums. It takes flexibility, moral rectitude, and a dedication to patient welfare as the top priority to overcome these obstacles.

Immunotherapy's unexplored possibilities present endless possibilities and the chance to treat illnesses that were previously thought to be incurable. But along with this potential is the moral responsibility to make sure that these treatments are created and implemented in an ethically sound and fair manner. Ethical standards will continue to be the cornerstone of the effort to harness the extraordinary potential of immunotherapy for the benefit of both individuals and society at large, even as science and technology progress.

CHAPTER 18
Immunotherapy's Ethical Frontier

One place on the path through the rapidly developing field of immunotherapy sticks out: the ethical frontier. This chapter explores the deep and frequently intricate ethical issues that come up in the field of immunotherapy.

Patient Independence:

The idea of patient autonomy is fundamental to immunotherapy. It represents people' rights to make knowledgeable decisions regarding their medical care. But as therapies grow more individualized and immunotherapy raises ethical questions beyond curing disease, people may be faced with previously unthinkable decisions. A major issue in the ethical frontier is striking a balance between the autonomy of the patient and the moral consequences of these decisions.

Non-maleficence and Beneficence:

Immunotherapy development and use are heavily influenced by the ethical precepts of beneficence (doing what is best for the patient) and non-maleficence (avoiding harm). An persistent ethical conundrum is balancing the interests of limiting damage and maximizing gains. It is a fine ethical tightrope to tread while ensuring that patients receive the most individualized and effective treatments while safeguarding their wellbeing.

Equity and Justice:

Justice as an ethical ideal places a strong emphasis on equity and just access to resources. It is morally necessary to make sure that all patients, regardless of socioeconomic background or geographic location, have access to these cutting-edge immunotherapy medicines. It will be crucial to address global health disparities and promote fair access to these treatments.

Security and Privacy of Data:

Immunotherapy requires large amounts of patient data, so data security and privacy become crucial ethical issues. It is ethically required to preserve sensitive data, have informed consent, and put strict data protection mechanisms in place. For these therapies to be effective, patients must believe that their data is handled ethically.

Improvement and Limitations:

Immunotherapy is pushing the ethical envelope and challenging social standards. Concerns concerning the ethical application of biotechnologies for non-medical uses surface as the field develops and has the potential to improve human immunity beyond the treatment of disease. In order to traverse these difficult challenges while respecting beneficence, non-maleficence, and autonomy, ethical discourse will be required.

Algorithms and Ethics in AI:

Artificial intelligence (AI) is a significant player in the immunotherapy ethical landscape. Treatment decisions are guided by AI-driven algorithms, which raises ethical concerns about their application in clinical settings. Transparency and ethical supervision are necessary to guarantee that AI improves medical care while upholding moral precepts like beneficence, non-maleficence, and patient autonomy.

Narratives of Patients and Empowerment:

Success tales from patients with immunotherapy have the ability to influence ethical thinking and inspire others. By telling these stories, we can promote patient-centered care and inspire optimism and resiliency. The value of patient narratives in campaigns to raise awareness and educate will be emphasized by ethical values.

International Cooperation and Ethical Alliances:

171

International cooperation is necessary to promote universal access to immunotherapy and address global health inequities. These initiatives will be led by ethical partnerships that prioritize the values of beneficence and justice. In order to achieve ethical healthcare parity, cooperation between governments, NGOs, and pharmaceutical firms will be essential.

Instruction and Knowledgeable Consent:

Informed consent and education are crucial at the ethical frontier. Patients are better able to make decisions consistent with their values when they are fully educated about all of their treatment options, including ethical issues. The significance of education and informed consent is emphasized by the ethical principles of beneficence and patient autonomy.

Ethical Supervision and Law:

Immunotherapy requires strict ethical supervision and control going forward. In order to guarantee that ethical standards are respected in clinical trials, therapy, and research, regulatory agencies and groups will be crucial. Patient safety, data privacy, and equal access to therapies are all included under ethical oversight.

Progress and Ethics in Balance:

The delicate balance between scientific advancement and ethical issues is being tested by the ethical frontier of immunotherapy. The responsible development and implementation of these innovative therapies will be guided by ethical standards, acting as a compass. An harmonious balance between advancement and moral considerations will be essential to the ethical frontier.

Immunotherapy's ethical frontier is a dynamic field characterized by changing social norms, scientific discoveries, and ethical standards.

Ethical principles will be the cornerstone for responsible and patient-centered advances as the sector grows, guaranteeing that these amazing cures are created and implemented in accordance with the strictest ethical guidelines.

Patient Independence:

A fundamental component of medical ethics is patient autonomy, which gives people the freedom to choose their healthcare providers based on information they have. Immunotherapy is an area in which this ethical principle assumes new relevance. Patients may have to make difficult decisions as therapies become more individualized and the ethical issues surrounding immunotherapy go beyond curing illness. These could involve taking part in clinical trials for novel medicines or strengthening their immune system for non-medical reasons. The extent to which patient autonomy should be honored and the best way to give them the knowledge they need to make these important decisions raise ethical concerns. Patients' opinions must be heard, and ethical frameworks must guarantee that they are adequately educated about the advantages, disadvantages, and ethical ramifications of any decisions they make.

Non-maleficence and Beneficence:

The research and application of immunotherapy are fundamentally guided by the ethical precepts of beneficence and non-maleficence. It can be difficult to strike the correct balance between maximizing advantages and limiting disadvantages. In order to protect patients' wellbeing, researchers and medical experts work to guarantee that they receive the most individualized and effective therapies possible. Deciding on the best course of therapy for patients might provide ethical challenges, especially when considering combination medicines. A thoughtful approach to treatment decisions is required by the ethical frontier, with a focus on doing what is most beneficial for the patient while inflicting the least amount of harm.

Equity and Justice:

As a moral precept, justice emphasizes the significance of equity and just access to resources. To achieve justice in the field of immunotherapy, all patients should have access to these cutting-edge medicines, irrespective of their geographic location or socioeconomic standing. This ethical consideration encompasses pushing for equal access to these medications and addressing global health disparities. It emphasizes the moral duty to make sure that patients in every part of the world have access to these transformative therapies. International attempts to attain healthcare fairness will be largely guided by ethical frameworks.

Security and Privacy of Data:

Since immunotherapy significantly depends on the gathering and evaluation of patient data, data security and privacy are vital ethical issues. It is morally required to protect private medical data. Patients need to have faith that their information is handled sensibly and privately. Maintaining patient confidence and ensuring the ethical use of patient data in research and treatment requires both adopting strict data protection measures and obtaining informed consent for data collection. In this field, ethical supervision is essential to maintaining patient privacy and security.

Improvement and Limitations:

Immunotherapy's ethical frontier questions accepted social mores and moral limits. Ethical concerns surface as the field develops to maybe improve the human immune system for uses other than medicine. These include questions about equity, safety, and the proper application of biotechnologies to transform the human situation. Ethical considerations such as beneficence, non-maleficence, and autonomy must be taken into account when discussing immune system improvement for longevity, performance, and resilience.

177

Algorithms and Ethics in AI:

The ethical frontier of immunotherapy is seeing a significant increase in the use of artificial intelligence (AI). Treatment decisions are made using machine learning algorithms, which raises ethical concerns about its application in clinical settings. It is crucial to make sure AI improves patient care while upholding moral precepts like beneficence, non-maleficence, and patient autonomy. Guidelines for preventing prejudice and discrimination in AI-driven healthcare decisions as well as ensuring that AI enhances rather than compromises patient well-being will be part of ethical oversight.

Narratives of Patients and Empowerment:

Success stories from patients receiving immunotherapy serve as both inspiration and platforms for moral advocacy. These stories can inspire others by highlighting the value of patient-centered care and the advantages of customized therapies. The importance of patient stories in education and awareness campaigns is highlighted by ethical standards. By promoting the ideals of hope, resiliency, and patient empowerment, sharing these stories helps people become knowledgeable and morally conscious citizens.

International Cooperation and Ethical Alliances:

In order to provide universal access to immunotherapy and address global health inequities, international collaboration must be driven by ethical concepts of beneficence and fairness. Achieving fair access to cutting-edge treatments will need cooperation between governments, nonprofits, and pharmaceutical firms. The ethical frontier emphasizes the moral need to make sure that all patients, no matter where they live, have access to these ground-breaking treatments, promoting global health fairness as a primary ethical objective.

Instruction and Knowledgeable Consent:

179

Informed consent and education are essential in the ethical field of immunotherapy. Patients need to be fully aware of all of their treatment options, including the moral implications of some therapies. Principles of ethics like beneficence and patient autonomy emphasize the value of education and informed consent in empowering people to make decisions that are in line with their values and best interests.

Ethical Supervision and Law:

Strong ethical control and regulation will be necessary for immunotherapy in the future to guarantee that moral principles are respected in clinical trials, treatment, and research. Ethical supervision will cover topics including fair access to therapies, patient safety, and data protection. In order to safeguard patient welfare and preserve public confidence in the advancement and use of immunotherapy, ethical regulation is necessary.

Progress and Ethics in Balance:

The ethical frontier calls into question the harmony between advancements in science and moral principles. These novel medicines are developed and implemented responsibly thanks to the compass provided by ethical standards. Navigating the immunotherapy's ethical frontier will require finding a balance between advancement and moral considerations. In order to guarantee that research and technology progress ethically and in the greatest interests of patient well-being, ethical frameworks will continue to change.

CHAPTER 19
The Development of Immunotherapy in Healthcare

Immunotherapy is leading the way in a revolutionary change in the medical field. The impact of immunotherapy on the development of healthcare—from diagnosis to treatment and beyond—is examined in this chapter.

Early Detection and Intervention:

The diagnosis and prevention of diseases are being redefined by immunotherapy. Early diagnosis of diseases including cancer and autoimmune disorders is now possible because to the use of immune system markers and genetic profiling. The adoption of early diagnosis has the potential to transform preventive and intervention techniques, leading to better patient outcomes and lower healthcare expenses in the long run.

Customized Medical Care:

A major factor propelling the era of personalized medicine is immunotherapy. By customizing care to each patient's distinct genetic and immunological composition, it maximizes effectiveness while reducing side effects. By putting more emphasis on patient-centric care rather than one-size-fits-all therapies, this strategy is changing the healthcare industry. Patients now actively participate in creating their own treatment programs rather than being passive beneficiaries of medical care.

Specialized Treatments:

Targeted therapeutic development is being driven by immunotherapy. The goal of these treatments is to spare healthy tissues while precisely targeting infections or sick cells. This accuracy not only increases the effectiveness of treatment but also lessens the side effects that are frequently connected to conventional treatments like radiation and chemotherapy.

Interprofessional Cooperation:

The effectiveness of immunotherapy depends on interdisciplinary cooperation between data analysts, geneticists, physicians, and scientists. The field of healthcare has evolved to adopt a more collaborative approach, realizing that complicated medical problems necessitate multidimensional solutions. The advancement of immunotherapy and healthcare in general depends heavily on this collaboration.

Developing New Therapeutic Pathways:

The treatment landscape is becoming more expansive as immunotherapy is being used to more disease domains. Once-untreatable conditions are being reevaluated, and novel treatments are beginning to surface. Diversifying treatment options could potentially address a variety of illnesses, including neurodegenerative problems, autoimmune disorders, and infectious infections.

Difficulties with Cost and Availability:

Despite the enormous potential of immunotherapy, issues with pricing and accessibility still exist. Navigating these challenges is part of the evolution of healthcare, since the high cost of certain immunotherapies raises concerns about equal access. Ensuring that all patients, irrespective of their socioeconomic condition, have access to these innovative treatments is an ethical challenge for policymakers and healthcare practitioners.

Healthcare Driven by Data:

Since immunotherapy requires a great deal of patient data, data-driven healthcare is becoming more and more prevalent. For the purpose of forecasting treatment results, spotting possible adverse effects, and streamlining therapeutic regimens, data analytics, artificial intelligence, and machine learning are essential. Healthcare is becoming more accurate, patient-centered, and efficient thanks to this data-driven approach.

Considering Ethics:

Ethics continue to be the most important factor as immunotherapy redefines healthcare. In order to address concerns like patient autonomy, beneficence, data privacy, and equal access, the ethical landscape of healthcare is changing. Immunotherapy is being developed and used responsibly thanks to the guidance of healthcare ethics.

International Health and Joint Research:

Immunotherapy has brought attention to how crucial international cooperation is in the medical field. The advancement of healthcare entails a dedication to tackling worldwide health inequalities and advocating for equitable access to cutting-edge treatments. International boundaries are being broken down by collaborative research, which emphasizes the moral values of beneficence and fairness.

Patient-First Healthcare:

Patient-centered treatment is increasingly becoming the norm because to immunotherapy. Patients are given the authority to speak up for themselves, share their experiences, and actively participate in healthcare choices. The ethical values of autonomy, beneficence, and non-maleficence are highlighted by the patient's voice, which has been a driving force behind the evolution of healthcare.

The development of immunotherapy is closely tied to the history of healthcare. This revolutionary method is impacting interdisciplinary cooperation, individualized medicine, and early diagnosis. Healthcare must address issues of affordability and accessibility while adhering to ethical principles as it develops. Patient autonomy, fairness, and beneficence will lead the worldwide partnership that characterizes the patient-centered, data-driven healthcare of the future.

Early Detection and Intervention:

Immunotherapy is pushing the envelope on early diagnosis and prevention, which is radically changing the healthcare environment. In the past, healthcare has been reactionary, with treatments frequently starting after illnesses have advanced noticeably. The focus of immunotherapy on genetics and the immune system has made it possible to diagnose patients earlier and with greater accuracy. Genetic profiling and biomarkers can detect diseases like cancer in their early stages, even before symptoms appear. This shift has the potential to completely reinterpret the meaning of prevention by making it possible to catch illnesses in the most curable stages. The trend toward early diagnosis holds promise for improving population health overall, saving lives, and lowering healthcare expenses.

Customized Medical Care:

In the age of customized medicine, immunotherapy is at the forefront, transforming both the experience and the delivery of healthcare. Treatments based on the individual genetic and immunological composition of each patient are replacing the conventional one-size-fits-all strategy. Patients now have more authority and are at the heart of their medical journey thanks to the transition from a generic to a highly individualized healthcare model. It highlights the significance of shared decision-making and informed consent, empowering patients to actively participate in creating their own treatment regimens. The shift in healthcare toward personalized medicine guarantees more patient-centered and efficacious therapies.

Specialized Treatments:

The development of highly tailored medicines is being led by immunotherapy. These medications are designed to precisely target infections or cells linked to disease, sparing healthy organs. This precision reduces the collateral damage that has been a problem with conventional therapies like radiation and chemotherapy, which is a huge advancement in healthcare. By reducing side effects, it improves the patient's quality of life in addition to increasing the effectiveness of the therapy. This development is evidence of the ongoing progress in healthcare, which is supported by advances in medical technology and scientific knowledge.

Interprofessional Cooperation:

The effectiveness of immunotherapy has shown how important interdisciplinary teamwork is in the medical field. Healthcare disciplines are dismantling their silos as a result of the need for comprehensive answers to complex medical problems. To fully realize the promise of immunotherapy, scientists, physicians, geneticists, and data analysts are collaborating. The healthcare industry's established hierarchy is being challenged by this collaborative approach, which also emphasizes the value of integrating different fields of knowledge and fosters teamwork. A new era of healthcare innovation and problem-solving is anticipated to be ushered in by the acceleration of the trend towards interdisciplinary collaboration as healthcare continues to change.

Developing New Therapeutic Pathways:

The therapeutic landscape is expanding as immunotherapy is being applied to previously untreatable disease domains. In light of immunotherapy's achievements, diseases that were previously thought to be incurable—such as some infectious diseases and neurodegenerative conditions—are now being reexamined. The advancement of healthcare is broadening the scope of available treatments, providing hope to those with illnesses for which there are few or no available treatments. Healthcare professionals, researchers, and legislators will need to negotiate the ethical challenges posed by these novel treatments as they develop.

Difficulties with Cost and Availability:

Immunotherapy has great potential, but it has also highlighted serious issues with pricing and accessibility. Serious concerns over fair access have been brought up by the exorbitant cost of certain immunotherapies. These concerns must be addressed in light of the evolution of healthcare, with a focus on guaranteeing that all patients, regardless of socioeconomic background, have access to these ground-breaking therapies. To make these life-saving treatments accessible to a larger population, legislators and healthcare professionals must confront the moral challenge of striking a balance between innovation and affordability.

Healthcare Driven by Data:

The need for large amounts of patient data for immunotherapy is driving the transition to data-driven healthcare. The way healthcare decisions are made is changing due to the combination of machine learning, artificial intelligence, and data analytics. Predictive algorithms are able to anticipate treatment results, recognize possible side effects, and tailor treatment plans. This data-driven strategy advances precision medicine, which improves patient outcomes, while also increasing the effectiveness of healthcare delivery. Data-driven healthcare promises to make healthcare more precise, patient-centered, and economical as it continues to change.

Considering Ethics:

The development of immunotherapy highlights difficult moral issues that are essential to the advancement of medical science. These ethical considerations include equitable access, data privacy, beneficence, and patient autonomy. The appropriate research and application of immunotherapy are guided by healthcare ethics, which guarantee that patient welfare is always the primary consideration in decision-making. Ethical standards offer a moral compass to navigate the benefits and challenges presented by these breakthrough cures as the healthcare landscape changes.

International Health and Joint Research:

Immunotherapy has highlighted the value of international cooperation in the medical field. The advancement of healthcare entails a dedication to tackling worldwide health inequalities and advocating for equitable access to cutting-edge treatments. International boundaries are being broken down by collaborative research, where organizations and researchers collaborate to improve healthcare outcomes and advance medical knowledge. The ethical precepts of beneficence and fairness are reflected in this international collaboration, emphasizing our shared need to guarantee that medical advancements benefit people everywhere.

Patient-First Healthcare:

The success of immunotherapy is driving the shift in healthcare to a patient-centered model. Patients are given the authority to speak up for themselves, share their experiences, and actively participate in healthcare choices. This evolution is propelled by the patient's voice, which highlights the moral precepts of autonomy, beneficence, and non-maleficence. Patients are now partners in determining their own healthcare path rather as merely being beneficiaries of medical treatment because to this shift towards patient-centered care.

The development of immunotherapy is inextricably linked to the advancement of healthcare. Early diagnosis, tailored medicine, interdisciplinary collaboration, and other areas are being impacted by this revolutionary approach. Healthcare must address issues of affordability and accessibility while adhering to ethical principles as it develops. Patient autonomy, fairness, and beneficence will lead the worldwide partnership that characterizes the patient-centered, data-driven healthcare of the future.

CHAPTER 20
Immunotherapy's Promise and Difficulties Outside of Healthcare

Immunotherapy is a novel method that goes beyond traditional medical practice by using the body's immune system to fight illness. We examine the possible benefits and drawbacks of immunotherapy in a number of societal domains and aspects in this chapter.

Food Security and Agriculture:

In agriculture, immunotherapy has great potential. This could lead to the development of more disease-resistant crops and livestock through the adaptation of immunotherapeutic methods. This could lead to more ecologically friendly and sustainable agriculture by lowering the demand for chemical pesticides and antibiotics and increasing food security.

Defense Against Biological and Chemical Threats:

The concepts of immunotherapy can be modified to protect against chemical and biological dangers. Creating immunotherapeutic plans for quick reactions to chemical or bioterrorism strikes can improve national security. Here, striking a balance between being ready and using these tools responsibly is a difficulty.

Preservation of the Environment:

The conservation of the environment may benefit from immunotherapy. It is feasible to lessen the risks related to biodiversity loss by using immune system principles to shield endangered animals from illnesses or invasive viruses. On the other hand, the possible effects on ecosystems and natural equilibriums are ethical considerations.

Addiction to Substances and Drugs:

Potential treatments for drug and substance addiction include immunotherapy. Creating vaccinations that trigger the body's defenses against chemicals that are addictive could help people recover from addiction. However, using immunotherapy for punitive rather than rehabilitative purposes raises ethical concerns.

Non-Medical Supplementation:

Immunotherapy raises the possibility of non-medical enhancement because of its capacity to treat diseases. There are moral and social issues when it comes to boosting the human immune system for things like increased lifespan, improved cognitive function, or improved physical performance. It can be quite difficult to strike the correct balance between society well-being and individual liberties.

Considerations for Ethics and Biosecurity:

When immunotherapy is used outside of the healthcare industry, biosecurity becomes critical.

Robust ethical and regulatory frameworks are necessary to ensure that immunotherapeutic technologies are not abused for malevolent ends. To avoid unintentional harm, these frameworks have to respect the concepts of responsible innovation, accountability, and international cooperation.

Awareness and Education of the Public:

Comprehensive public education and awareness initiatives are necessary to expand the use of immunotherapy outside of the healthcare industry. It is imperative that society is apprised of the possible advantages, hazards, and ethical implications associated with these innovative uses. Informed decision-making and the proper use of immunotherapeutic technology require public interaction.

Working Together Internationally:

When immunotherapy is used for purposes other than healthcare, international cooperation becomes essential. In research and applications, ethical relationships, norms, and agreements are essential to guarantee responsible use and avoid power imbalances. Additionally, international cooperation can assist in addressing the global issues raised by immunotherapy's non-medical uses.

Control & Supervision:

Immunotherapy non-medical applications regulation is a difficult task. It calls for the creation of precise rules, regulations, and supervision systems. Finding a balance between promoting innovation and guarding against abuse is a difficult task.

The Role of Society and Ethical Limits:

The use of immunotherapy outside of the healthcare industry emphasizes the necessity of moral limits and community involvement. It is up to society to define these limits and make sure that immunotherapy is used responsibly in a way that is consistent with its ethics, values, and long-term health.

Immunotherapy has the ability to address a wide range of possibilities and issues in a variety of sectors as it expands outside healthcare. To maximize their promise while reducing hazards, these technologies must be used responsibly, which calls for ethical concerns, legal frameworks, and social involvement. The expansion of immunotherapy's use beyond medicine is evidence of the unbounded potential of scientific advancement, where a moral compass is crucial for navigating unexplored territory.

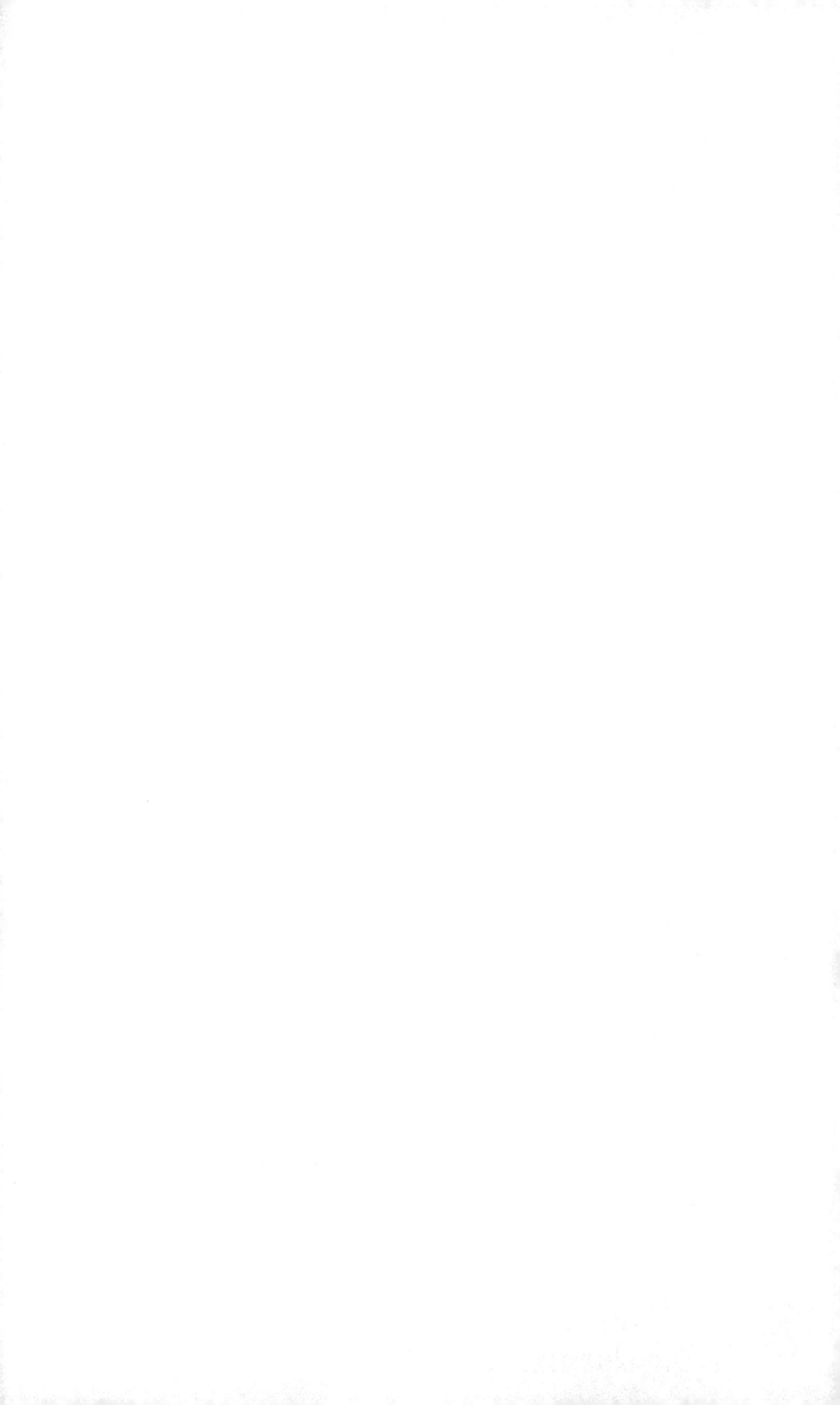